ESSENTIALS for
the **A&E NURSE**

Jennifer R. Buettner, BSN, RN, CEN, currently serves as an education coordinator for the A&E at Emory Hillandale Hospital in the Atlanta, Georgia, area. In this role, Mrs. Buettner works to advance the careers of emergency nurses through education and evidence-based practice. She finds great joy in helping others grow professionally and cultivate their inner gifts and talents. She has developed A&E orientation processes and education courses for several local hospitals in the Atlanta area. In her 22 years of A&E nursing experience, she has spent several years precepting new emergency nurses and has served as a legal nurse consultant. Mrs. Buettner holds certifications in basic disaster life support (BDLS) and advanced disaster life support (ADLS), is a certified emergency nurse (CEN), and serves as an advanced cardiovascular life support (ACLS), pediatric advanced life support (PALS), and CPR instructor. She is a course coordinator for the trauma nursing core course (TNCC) and emergency nursing pediatric course (ENPC). She is a current member of the Emergency Nurses Association and an advocate for the Board Certification for Emergency Nursing. She received the Faculty Award from the Virginia Beach School of Practical Nursing, for the graduate who "has achieved excellence in both the academic and clinical settings and who best exemplifies the total integration of program philosophy to professional performance" (March 1999). In 2010, Mrs. Buettner was nominated as the nurse of the year by the *Atlanta Journal-Constitution*. She was a finalist for the 2016 Atlanta March of Dimes' Nurse of the Year Award. Her passion to teach and mentor new A&E nurses led her to create an original A&E orientation manual made specifically for new emergency nurses and their preceptors.

OTHER *ESSENTIALS* BOOKS

Essentials for the **A&E NURSE**: Guide to a Successful Accident and Emergency Department Orientation, Fourth Edition *(Buettner)*

Essentials on **ADOLESCENT HEALTH FOR NURSING AND HEALTH PROFESSIONALS**: A Care Guide *(Herrman)*

Essentials for the **ADULT-GERONTOLOGY ACUTE CARE NURSE PRACTITIONER** *(Carpenter)*

Essentials for the **ANTEPARTUM AND POSTPARTUM NURSE**: A Nursing Orientation and Care Guide *(Davidson)*

Essentials Workbook for **CARDIAC DYSRHYTHMIAS AND 12-LEAD EKGs** *(Desmarais)*

Essentials for the **CARDIAC SURGERY NURSE**: Caring for Cardiac Surgery Patients, Third Edition *(Hodge)*

Essentials for **CAREER SUCCESS IN NURSING**: Making the Most of Mentoring *(Vance)*

Essentials for the **CATH LAB NURSE** *(McCulloch)*

Essentials for the **CLASSROOM NURSING INSTRUCTOR**: Classroom Teaching *(Yoder-Wise, Kowalski)*

Essentials for the **CLINICAL NURSE LEADER** *(Wilcox, Deerhake)*

Essentials for the **CLINICAL NURSE MANAGER**: Managing a Changing Workplace, Second Edition *(Fry)*

Essentials for the **CLINICAL NURSING INSTRUCTOR**: Clinical Teaching, Third Edition *(Kan, Stabler-Haas)*

Essentials on **COMBATING NURSE BULLYING, INCIVILITY, AND WORKPLACE VIOLENCE**: What Nurses Need to Know *(Ciocco)*

Essentials About **COMPETENCY-BASED EDUCATION IN NURSING**: How to Teach Competency Mastery *(Wittmann-Price, Gittings)*

Essentials for the **CRITICAL CARE NURSE**, Second Edition *(Hewett)*

Essentials About **CURRICULUM DEVELOPMENT IN NURSING**: How to Develop and Evaluate Educational Programs, Second Edition *(McCoy, Anema)*

Essentials for **DEMENTIA CARE**: What Nurses Need to Know, Second Edition *(Miller)*

Essentials for **DEVELOPING A NURSING ACADEMIC PORTFOLIO**: What You Really Need to Know *(Wittmann-Price)*

Essentials for **DNP ROLE DEVELOPMENT**: A Career Navigation Guide *(Menonna-Quinn, Tortorella Genova)*

Essentials About **EKGs FOR NURSES**: The Rules of Identifying EKGs *(Landrum)*

Essentials for **EVIDENCE-BASED PRACTICE IN NURSING**: Third Edition *(Godshall)*

Essentials for the **FAITH COMMUNITY NURSE**: Implementing FCN/Parish Nursing *(Hickman)*

Essentials About **FORENSIC NURSING**: What You Need to Know *(Scannell)*

Essentials for the **GERONTOLOGY NURSE**: A Nursing Care Guide *(Eliopoulos)*

Essentials About **GI AND LIVER DISEASES FOR NURSES**: What APRNs Need to Know *(Chaney)*

Essentials About the **GYNECOLOGICAL EXAM**: A Professional Guide for NPs, PAs, and Midwives, Second Edition *(Secor, Fantasia)*

Essentials in **HEALTH INFORMATICS FOR NURSES** *(Hardy)*

Essentials for **HEALTH PROMOTION IN NURSING**: Promoting Wellness *(Miller)*

Essentials for Nurses About **HOME INFUSION THERAPY**: The Expert's Best Practice Guide *(Gorski)*

Essentials for the **HOSPICE NURSE**: A Concise Guide to End-of-Life Care, Second Edition *(Wright)*

Essentials for the **L&D NURSE**: Labor & Delivery Orientation, Second Edition *(Groll)*

Essentials About **LBGTQ+ CARE FOR NURSES** *(Traister)*

Essentials for the **LONG-TERM CARE NURSE**: What Nursing Home and Assisted Living Nurses Need to Know *(Eliopoulos)*

Essentials to **LOVING YOUR RESEARCH PROJECT**: A Stress-Free Guide for Novice Researchers in Nursing and Healthcare *(Marshall)*

Essentials for **MAKING THE MOST OF YOUR CAREER IN NURSING** *(Redulla)*

Essentials for **MANAGING PATIENTS WITH A PSYCHIATRIC DISORDER**: What RNs, NPs, and New Psych Nurses Need to Know *(Marshall)*

Essentials About **MEDICAL CANNABIS AND OPIOIDS**: Minimizing Opioid Use Through Cannabis *(Smith, Smith)*

Essentials for the **MEDICAL OFFICE NURSE**: What You Really Need to Know *(Richmeier)*

Essentials for the **MEDICAL–SURGICAL NURSE**: Clinical Orientation *(Ciocco)*

ESSENTIALS for the **A&E NURSE**

Guide to a Successful Accident and Emergency Department Orientation

Fourth Edition

Jennifer R. Buettner, BSN, RN, CEN

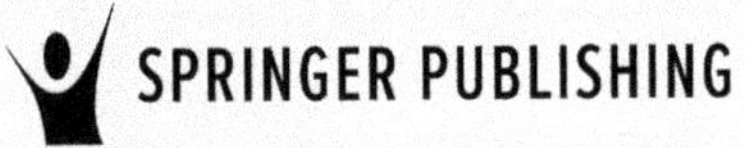

Springer Publishing Company, LLC
11 West 42nd Street, New York, NY 10036
www.springerpub.com
connect.springerpub.com/

Acquisitions Editor: Elizabeth Nieginski
Compositor: Amnet Systems

ISBN: 978-0-8261-6715-6

The author and the publisher of this Work have made every effort to use sources believed to be reliable to provide information that is accurate and compatible with the standards generally accepted at the time of publication. Because medical science is continually advancing, our knowledge base continues to expand. Therefore, as new information becomes available, changes in procedures become necessary. We recommend that the reader always consult current research and specific institutional policies before performing any clinical procedure or delivering any medication. The author and publisher shall not be liable for any special, consequential, or exemplary damages resulting, in whole or in part, from the readers' use of, or reliance on, the information contained in this book. The publisher has no responsibility for the persistence or accuracy of URLs for external or third-party Internet websites referred to in this publication and does not guarantee that any content on such websites is, or will remain, accurate or appropriate.

The *Essentials* series was published in the United States of America as the *Fast Facts* series.

This book is dedicated to A&E nurses everywhere.
May these pages provide you a strong foundation of knowledge and wisdom.
Let your cups overflow with strength, grace, compassion, mercy, and love.
May God bless your hearts and hands as you touch
so many people in need each and every day.

Contents

Reviewers of the Fourth Edition

Reviewers of the Previous Edition

Natasha Allen, RN, CEN
R. Bruce Bessey, MD, FAAP
Theresa M. Campo, DNP, RN, NP-C
Nancy Capponi, MSN, RN, CEN, CCRN
Joanne Davis, DMD
Kurtis Davis, DMD
Julie Espinosa, MSN, RN, CEN, EMT-P
Paula Funderburke, MS, RN, CEN, CPEN, CNS-BC
Cyndi Griffith, BSN, RN
Heather Hall, MD
Shunda L. Harper, MSN, RN
Nichole Lunsford Howell, BSN, RN
Chanique Kelley, MSN, RN, CEN
Paul Olander, MSW, JD, LCSW, CCM, NBCCH, RRT-P
Laura K. Phillips, MSN, RN
Joshua W. Shoemaker, PharmD, BCPS
Tamiko Smith, MSN, FNP-C
Sealena White, BSN, RN

Preface

This is a book designed for *real* A&E nurses by a *real* A&E nurse. It is a book for quick reference intended to aid your day-to-day A&E orientation process with your preceptor and to guide you through the *most common illnesses* seen in the A&E. This book does not cover basic anatomy and physiology, advanced practice emergency medicine, advanced cardiovascular life support, pediatric advanced life support, or the trauma nurse core course. The information in this book has been compiled from basic A&E knowledge, and the references used are considered reliable.

There are several points to take into consideration in referencing this book. First, interventions listed that go beyond the scope of nursing practice should be followed as ordered by the A&E provider. Second, the term "provider" in this book could refer to a physician (MD or DO), a nurse practitioner (NP), or a physician assistant (PA) who is qualified to provide such A&E patient care. In most cases, interventions that go beyond the usual scope of nursing practice have been introduced using "Anticipate an order to," followed by a list of possible provider orders. As always, it is the nurse's responsibility to check any noted medication dosages or treatments to ensure that all are current, recommended, and accepted practices.

After reading this book, you will become the "Jack of all illnesses." Therefore, put on your running shoes, keep a stash of dark chocolates, and, when all else fails, practice unreasonable happiness. One thing is for sure: Just when you think you have seen it all, your next patient will come in!

Each chapter includes a brief introduction; an outline of materials, equipment, and drugs with which you should become familiar; a list of diagnoses that includes definitions, causes, signs and symptoms, and interventions; a feature titled Essentials that provides quick summaries of important points; and question-and-answer boxes for your review. The appendices at the end of the book include abbreviations, skills checklists, IV drips, common lab values, EKG rhythms, and frequently used A&E medications—information that should become second nature to all A&E personnel.

Jennifer R. Buettner

Acknowledgments

I could not do what I do without the support of my loving husband, Nick, and our friends and family. Nevertheless, the base of my emergency nursing foundation was built by my first preceptor, Linda Whitt, BSN, RN. I thank her for her patience, sharing her wealth of knowledge, and setting a prime example of a truly humble, wise, and compassionate nurse. I cannot forget my second preceptor, Walter McCracken, RN, whose pearls of wisdom can be found in no book. Special thanks go to my editor, Elizabeth Nieginski; assistant editor, Hannah Hicks; and the Springer Publishing team for bringing my thoughts and ideas for this book to life. I would like to acknowledge the work of the reviewers of both this edition and the previous editions in offering their professional opinions and reviewing the content in this book for accuracy. I am truly honored to be a part of a dedicated, knowledgeable, and compassionate A&E leadership team, including Michael Steele, MSN, RN, CEN; Eva Williams, BSN, RN; and Natasha Allen, FNP, RN, CEN—I thank you for mentoring, supporting, and inspiring me even on my weakest days! To all my friends and colleagues who have inspired me and molded me into the A&E nurse I am today, I am forever grateful.

Last, but not least, I would like to thank the nurse and good friend who inspired me to write this book and never stopped believing in me: Nichole Lunsford Howell, BSN, RN.

Above all, my faith has sustained me through all my endeavors; I give thanks and glory to God for all of His gifts and blessings.

1

Tips on Surviving A&E Nursing

Even if you love working in the A&E, it can be tough at times. The A&E is particularly stressful because you care for a broad spectrum of patients in a fast-paced, critical environment. So, you not only need to be extremely knowledgeable but also need to be organized, calm, and fast on your feet. Everyone knows that the nurses are the very heart of the A&E. Your patients rely on you. But **to take care of others, you first need to *practice self-care,*** physically, mentally, and spiritually. This chapter includes a checklist of stress symptoms and a list of simple methods for coping with those pressures.

During this part of your orientation, locate and become familiar with:

- How to recognize the symptoms of stress on the job
- Basic techniques you can use on the job to alleviate that stress

SYMPTOMS OF STRESS

It is true that A&E nurses are sometimes referred to as "adrenaline junkies." However, one cannot function on adrenaline alone. Severe stress and anxiety on the job are harmful to you and your patients. So learn to recognize the signs and symptoms: severe muscle tension, fatigue, irritability, flight or fight response, tachycardia, tachypnea, weakness, sweating, feeling helpless, anger, tearfulness, urinary urgency, diarrhea, dry mouth, insomnia, difficulty in problem-solving, feeling overwhelmed, and decreased appetite.

Notes: ____

____

____

____

____

____

____

____

____

____

____

____

____

____

____

____

Essential Facts

To take care of others well, you first need to take care of yourself.

TECHNIQUES FOR RELIEVING STRESS

- Take a moment, close your eyes, and take some deep cleansing abdominal breaths. Breathe in through your nose as you count to 5. Then exhale slowly through your mouth as you count to 5, and that's it. Breathing exercises increase oxygen to your brain and are a fast, simple way to relieve stress anytime, anywhere. Since you have to wash your hands for 20 seconds, try doing it twice every time you wash your hands.
- Stay hydrated. Keep a water bottle with you at work in an approved designated area. Staying hydrated is an easy way to stay healthy.
- Focus on the positives. Optimism may not come naturally, but it is a behavior that can be learned. Resiliency skills can be built. Practice it over and over again until it becomes a habit (about 30 days). Your brain can be retrained. Reframe any negative statements into positive ones. Practice positive self-talk every morning in the mirror. Choose gratitude and joy daily. Change your thinking; change your life! When you have a complaint, spend your energy finding a solution rather than complaining. As a nurse, you need all the energy you can get, so use it to resolve stressful problems.
- Prioritize time in your regular work week for rest and rejuvenation. Consider ways to rest and recharge physically, mentally, and spiritually throughout the week. Schedule vacations at least annually. Schedule time to work out, pray, go to church, journal, and talk with a trusted friend or counselor.
- Listen to upbeat energizing music on the way to work so that the melody will repeat itself in your head all day. "Whistle while you work." Singing or humming is a good way to relieve stress.
- Keep a stash of healthy snacks and drinks or my personal favorite: *dark* chocolates. They are a source of energy and antioxidants. Dark chocolate not only boosts your immune system but also seems to make people happy. It works well on any grumpy coworkers too, so do not forget to share.
- Be proactive and keep your patients informed. Introduce yourself to patients and their family members when you enter a room and **establish goals with them**. Keeping patients and family members informed relieves their stress. Tell them who you are, what you are doing, and when it will happen. If you want to make a great impression, learn to anticipate your patient's needs and then go

the extra mile. Throw in unexpected extras like warmed blankets, pillows, cups of coffee (if allowed), prayer, or extra educational materials.

- Invest in a well-made, comfortable pair of shoes. Eight to 12 hours of painful swollen feet will only add to your stress.
- Recognize that it is perfectly normal to feel anxious during a code (e.g., cardiac/pulmonary arrest). Only time, practice, and training will help you cope with the anxiety felt when performing advanced cardiovascular life-supportive treatments.
- Do not think or act as if you know it all. Medicine is constantly changing. No matter how much A&E experience you have, you can still learn something new every day.
- Look for growth opportunities. Seek frequent feedback from your leaders and grab a cup of coffee and learn from other high-performing colleagues. Find what your leader's pet peeves are. What are their time management secrets or tips? I recommend *The Great Employee Handbook*.
- Keep the following in your pocket every day: trauma shears, hemostats, tape, pen, calculator (with list of A&E intravenous drips and doses taped to back), and this book. Being prepared will reduce stress and anxiety.
- Invest in a good pair of support socks or hose and do leg exercises. Most nurses eventually develop varicose veins. It is hard to take good care of your patients when your legs ache and have poor circulation.
- Ask or look up any medications about which you are unsure. There are numerous medication routes and doses to memorize. Looking them up in hospital-recommended software or asking colleagues will help you learn them and keep your patients safe and free of medication errors.
- Keep your uniforms clean, to save yourself the hassle of having to buy new scrubs frequently. Wash out Betadine (povidone-iodine) or benzoic stains on your scrubs with rubbing alcohol. Pour hydrogen peroxide on any blood spots on your uniform and let foam for a minute. Then wash with soap and cold water. You may want to keep an extra pair of scrubs in your locker or car.
- Learn how to talk respectfully to others by reading up on how to engage effectively in difficult conversations. About 80% of medical errors occur because of poor communication. I recommend the book *Crucial Conversations*. Accept constructive criticism. If you want to gain your peers respect, do not make excuses. Instead say, "I appreciate your feedback. What can I do to ensure this doesn't happen again?"

- Be a team player. Be the nurse you want to work with. Learn how to delegate tasks the right way.
- Enjoy your work and have a sense of humor, even if it seems unreasonable. You will not survive without one. Laughter is often the best medicine.
- Avoid gossip and any work-related posts on social media. Have you ever heard the phrase "nothing about me without me"? If someone is not present, then you should not be speaking about them. If you have an issue or question, resolve it by speaking directly to the person involved. We are all on the same team. We need to build each other up, not tear each other down. Build relationships with your colleagues. Take care of each other. Try writing a thank you card to one colleague per month. It is okay to seek advice on how to deal with certain situations; find a trustworthy, experienced mentor and have lunch with them.
- Increase your A&E knowledge. Join the Emergency Nurses Association, sign up for A&E-related courses, go to conferences, and study from a certified emergency nurse (CEN) review book. Ask for training. Increasing your knowledge base is key for better patient care.
- Maintain liability insurance on yourself. It is inexpensive, and the A&E is a very litigious area. Liability insurance is a simple way to protect yourself.
- Document, document, document! How was the patient when they came in? Document airway, breathing, circulation, and neurologic assessment findings. **Avoid shortcuts.** Develop good assessment skills early on and know that patients do not always present according to the textbook. Chart on your nonurgent patient about once every hour; on a critical patient, as frequent as every 5 to 10 minutes. Chart when you assumed care of the patient. Document how the patient was when he or she left the A&E (e.g., ambulatory, stable, age appropriate, alert) and reassess airway, breathing, and circulation (ABCs).

Notes: ____

Essential Facts

- Practice self-care by regularly scheduling time to address your spiritual, physical, and mental needs.
- Take care of each other.
- Document, document, document!

SUMMARY

Emergency nursing is not for everyone. It can be indescribably hard at times, and everyone experiences a bad day here and there. But if you practice these simple stress-relieving techniques, you will be able to survive whatever the A&E throws at you. If you can make it through the tough times, you will survive long enough to find out just how rewarding A&E nursing can be. After all, isn't that why you chose this profession in the first place?

2

Acid–Base Imbalances

The body requires a delicate balance of acids and bases to main-tain natural homeostasis. Many life-threatening illnesses affect the acid–base balance. Therefore, recognizing any acid–base imbalance is crucial to saving someone's life. As a nurse in the A&E, you will come across acid–base imbalances daily. Many new and experienced nurses find acid–base balance difficult to understand. After reviewing this chapter and learning the three simple steps provided, you will find it much easier to remember how to interpret test results. **Understanding the pathophysiology and reviewing many laboratory results are key to better understanding acid–base imbalances.**

During this part of your orientation, locate and become familiar with:

- Arterial or venous blood gas procedures and results
- Diabetic ketoacidosis protocols
- Intubation equipment
- Medications to know: insulin, sodium bicarbonate, potassium, and dextrose

Acid–base balance is controlled by two organ systems.

RESPIRATORY SYSTEM

You breathe in oxygen (O_2) and breathe out carbon dioxide (CO_2). In the bloodstream, CO_2 mixes with water (H_2O) to make carbonic acid (H_2CO_3).

Notes: ____

RENAL SYSTEM

H_2CO_3 dissociates into a base, a bicarbonate (HCO_3^-), and an acid (H^+), which is excreted or conserved by the kidneys. Normal pH of plasma contains a ratio of 20 bicarbonates to 1 carbonic acid.

Notes: ____

RECOGNIZING AN IMBALANCE

An easy way to remember whether your patient has a respiratory or metabolic imbalance, as shown in Table 2.1, is this simple mnemonic.

For pH/bicarbonate directions in acidosis versus alkalosis, remember **ROME:**

Respiratory is **O**pposite (pH and CO_2), **M**etabolic is **E**qual (pH and HCO_3^-)

Table 2.1

Determining Acid–Base Imbalances			
ABG	**pH**	**CO$_2$**	**HCO$_3^-$**
Respiratory acidosis	<7.35	↑	Normal or ↑
Respiratory alkalosis	>7.45	↓	Normal or ↓
Metabolic acidosis	<7.35	Normal or ↓	↓
Metabolic alkalosis	>7.45	Normal or ↑	↑

Normal pH = 7.35–7.45; normal $PaCO_2$ = 35–45; normal HCO_3^- = 22–26.

ABG, arterial blood gas; HCO_3^-, bicarbonate; $PaCO_2$, partial pressure of carbon dioxide.

The arrows in Table 2.1 for respiratory pH and partial pressure of arterial carbon dioxide ($PaCO_2$) are in opposite directions from each other, and the arrows for metabolic pH and bicarbonate point in the same direction.

Notes: ____

Essential Facts

Acid–base balance is controlled by the respiratory and renal systems.

Venous blood gases are typically 0.03 to 0.04 less than arterial blood gas values.

DIAGNOSES

Every acid–base imbalance is **described using three words**, such as uncompensated respiratory acidosis. To determine which imbalance your patient has, follow these three simple steps. Table 2.1 provides a visual guide of these steps.

1. Look at the pH. If it is normal (7.35–7.45), it is *compensated.* If it is out of range, it is *uncompensated.*
2. A pH <7.35 is *acidosis.* A pH >7.45 is *alkalosis.*
3. Look at $PaCO_2$ and HCO_3^-. Abnormal $PaCO_2$ = *respiratory.* Abnormal HCO_3^- = *metabolic.* If both are abnormal, it is both *respiratory* and *metabolic.*

RESPIRATORY ACIDOSIS

In respiratory acidosis, pH is <7.35 because of **inadequate ventilations.** Poor ventilation causes poor oxygenation and one to retain CO_2. That means O_2 cannot get in, and CO_2 cannot get out. CO_2 builds up and mixes with H_2O, resulting in H_2CO_3 lowering pH. HCO_3^- is normal. This patient is at risk for hypoxia.

- *Causes:* Upper airway obstruction; pulmonary edema; **hypoventilation**; head trauma; chest trauma; pneumonia; chronic obstructive pulmonary disease (COPD); narcotic overdose; and muscle weakness.
- *Signs and symptoms:* Tachycardia; headache; decreased pulse oximetry reading; increased end title CO_2 (etCO_2) > 45 mmHg;

confusion; weakness; coma; hyperkalemia; cyanosis; bradypnea; paralysis; and respiratory arrest.

- *Interventions:* Administer O_2; give nebulized breathing treatments; **treat underlying condition; prepare for intubation**; provide mechanical ventilation; measure pulse O_2; monitor cardiac rhythm; and obtain an intravenous access.

Notes: ____

Question: What supplies are needed to intubate a patient?
Answer: *High-flow O_2, suction, Ambu bag, appropriate size endotracheal tube, 10-mL syringe of air, stylet, appropriate blades (Miller/ Macintosh) with working handle, CO_2 detector or waveform capnography device, tape or endotracheal tube securing device, and stethoscope to check placement.*

RESPIRATORY ALKALOSIS

In respiratory alkalosis, pH is >7.45. When a person **hyperventilates**, they expel all of their CO_2. There is no CO_2 left to mix with H_2O to make H_2CO_3. No acid = alkalosis. HCO_3^- is normal.

- *Causes:* Hyperventilation; pain; anxiety; pulmonary embolus; hypoxia; high altitude; drug toxicity (early salicylate adult overdose); third-trimester pregnancy; and fever.
- *Signs and symptoms:* Tetany or seizures from hypocalcemia; **hypokalemia**, diaphoresis; tingling of extremities; decrease in end title CO_2 (etCO$_2$) < 35 mmHg; dizziness; altered mental status; anxiety; dyspnea; paresthesia; palpitations; tachycardia; and hyperventilation.
- *Interventions:* Encourage **slow deep breathing**; correct underlying condition; provide fluids intravenously; and **correct hyperventilation** with nonrebreather mask *without* O_2.

Notes: ____

Essential Facts

- Hyperventilation treatment: Put O_2 nonrebreather mask over the patient's face and leave turned off. (It works like a paper bag.)
- Salicylate (aspirin) poisoning increases CO_2 production and oxygen consumption resulting in respiratory alkalosis initially and in severe cases leads to renal damage and metabolic acidosis.
- The oxyhemoglobin dissociation curve demonstrates how changes in pH and/or body temperature directly impact oxygen affinity to hemoglobin (Figure 2.1). Acidosis and hyperthermia reduce oxyhemoglobin affinity, where alkalosis and hypothermia increase the tight bonds of oxyhemoglobin instead of exchanging with the peripheral tissues. Both can **result in poor oxygen exchange.**

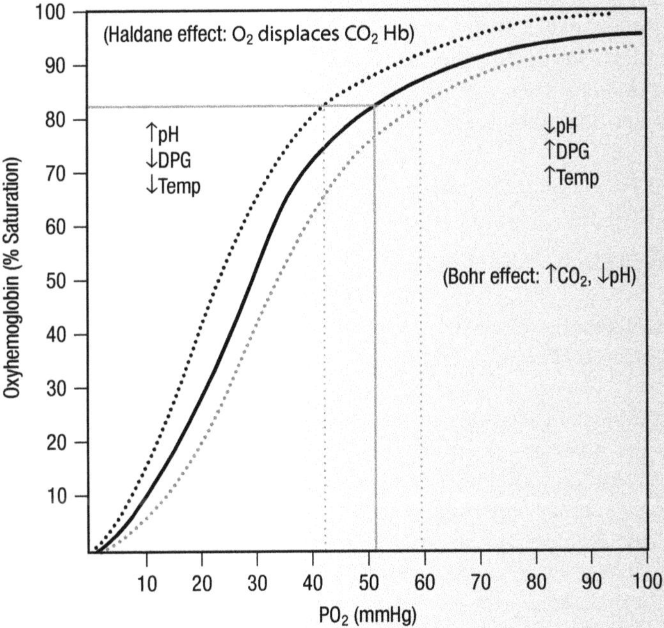

Figure 2.1 Oxyhemoglobin dissociation curve.

DPG, diphosphoglycerate.

Source: Ratznium.

METABOLIC ACIDOSIS

In metabolic acidosis, pH is <7.35 due to a decrease in HCO_3^- or increase in H^+ ion. $PaCO_2$ is normal. The kidneys compensate by excreting excess H^+ ions.

- *Causes:* **Diabetic ketoacidosis**; renal disease; starvation; hypothermia **shock** or **sepsis;** and loss of bicarbonate in severe diarrhea.
- *Signs and symptoms:* Altered mental state; hypotension; abdominal pain; nausea, vomiting, and diarrhea; Kussmaul respirations; **hyperventilation** as a compensatory mechanism; tingling and numbness; decreased $etCO_2$ < 35 mmHg; hyperkalemia; peaked T waves; flushed, warm skin; headache; bradycardia; and muscle weakness.
- *Interventions:* Provide fluids intravenously (lactated ringer's); treatment may include intravenous sodium bicarbonate, intravenous dextrose, and intravenous regular insulin (to put potassium back in cells); assist ventilations; monitor cardiac rhythm; and perform basic metabolic panel (BMP).

Notes: ____

METABOLIC ALKALOSIS

In metabolic alkalosis, the pH is >7.45 due to elevated HCO_3^- or decreased H^+. $PaCO_2$ is normal.

- *Causes:* Loss of stomach acid associated with **vomiting**; ingesting too many alkali substances (antacids, milk of magnesia, or baking soda); diuretics; **hypokalemia**; and Cushing's syndrome.
- *Signs and symptoms:* Hypocalcemia (tetany, twitching, irritability, shaking, and seizures); confusion; nausea, vomiting, and diarrhea; coma; decreased ST segment on EKG; bradypnea; hypokalemia (muscle weakness and loss of reflexes); and polyuria.
- *Interventions:* Anticipate orders to **prevent vomiting** with antiemetics, avoid gastric suctioning, administer normal saline intravenously, perform BMP, **provide potassium** supplements for hypokalemia, and monitor cardiac performance and respirations.

Notes: ____

Essential Facts

Here is a memory trick, with al**KaLO**sis, the serum **K** (potassium level) is **LO**w (hypokalemia).

The opposite is true in acidosis; the serum potassium is high (hyperkalemia).

Question: Before your patient has an arterial blood gas drawn, what test should be performed?

Answer: *Allen's test.*

SUMMARY

Although acid–base imbalances can be challenging to understand, they are critical to maintaining natural homeostasis. An A&E nurse comes across acid–base imbalances on a daily basis. Check your patient's arterial or venous blood gas results and anticipate interventions. **Practice** the steps provided in this chapter so you will be able to accurately interpret test results.

3

Cardiovascular Emergencies

In the A&E, cardiovascular diseases are an everyday life-threatening occurrence. However, **with proper assessment and fast treatment, cardiac diseases are resolved every day in A&Es** across the country. After studying this chapter, you will have a basic understanding of cardiovascular assessments and treatments. This chapter does not replace EKG courses or the advanced cardiovascular life support certification required to work in the A&E. **Many nurses find keeping an advanced cardiovascular life support handbook for study very helpful.**

During this part of your orientation, locate and become familiar with:

- EKGs and supplies
- ST-segment elevated myocardial infarction (STEMI) policy and protocol for your facility
- Advanced cardiovascular life support and EKG courses available to you
- Cardiac monitors, defibrillators, and pacers
- Crash carts
- Pacer magnets
- Medications to know: aspirin, alteplase, morphine, nitroglycerin, atropine, adenosine, digoxin, furosemide, calcium channel blockers, beta-blockers, amiodarone, lidocaine, epinephrine, vasopressin, heparin, warfarin, dopamine, nicardipine hydrochloride, and norepinephrine

CONGESTIVE HEART FAILURE

In congestive heart failure, the heart fails to pump blood effectively. It can be acute or chronic. As a result, blood backs up. It can back up to the body (right-sided congestive heart failure) or the lungs (left-sided congestive heart failure).

- *Causes:* Other illnesses can, over time, lead to congestive heart failure. These include hypertension; arrhythmias; diabetes; coronary artery disease; valvular stenosis; cardiomyopathy; emphysema; obesity; pulmonary embolism; anemia; and thyroid disease.
- *Signs and symptoms:*
    - *Right sided:* Pitting pedal edema; hepatojugular reflux; liver enlargement; nocturia; and jugular vein distention.
    - *Left sided:* Usually develops first; crackles; shortness of breath; pulmonary edema (rales); tachypnea; left ventricular hypertrophy; tachycardia; and ventricular gallop.
- *Interventions:* Use the mnemonic **UNLOAD FAST**. Anticipate orders for **U**pright position, **N**itroglycerin, **L**asix, **O**xygen, **A**ce inhibitors, **D**igoxin, **F**luid restrictions, **A**rterial blood gas (ABG), and **S**odium restrictions and **T**ests (digoxin levels, ABG, and metabolic panel). Also establish intravenous (IV) access; monitor cardiac performance; and monitor intake and output. Provide condom catheter, external female catheter, urinal, bedside commode, or bedpan for frequent urination after furosemide administration.

Notes: ____

____

____

____

____

____

____

Question: Which patient position is best to hear S3 (ventricular gallop) and S4 (atrial gallop)?
Answer: *Left lateral.*

ACUTE MYOCARDIAL INFARCTION

Acute myocardial infarction is the result of a clogged coronary artery supplying blood to the heart muscle. The patient's history often reveals hypertension, coronary artery disease, high cholesterol, and smoking (see Figure 3.1).

- *Causes:* Blood clots; coronary arterial spasm from cocaine use; contributing factors: hypertension; coronary artery disease; smoking; obesity; hyperlipidemia; and genetics.
- *Signs and symptoms:* Nausea and vomiting; diaphoresis; shortness of breath; fatigue; anxiety; hypertension or hypotension; and chest pain (described often as pressure, squeezing, tightness, or vague) that may radiate to the left shoulder or jaw. Females may present with vague weakness, fatigue, and dyspnea. EKG may or may not reveal ST segment elevation.
- *Interventions:* **MOVE!!** (**M**onitor, **O**xygen, **V**enous access [2 large bore], and **E**KG within 7 minutes); anticipate orders to administer medications **MONA** (**M**orphine, **O**xygen, **N**itroglycerin sublingual (SL), and **A**spirin); obtain cardiac enzymes; arrange for chest x-ray and cardiologist consult; prepare for possible **cardiac cath lab admission** or thrombolytics (alteplase), anticoagulant (heparin) therapy; and reassess/monitor chest pain.

Notes: ____

____

____

Question: What factors absolutely contraindicate the use of thrombolytics?
Answer: *Active bleeding, recent surgery, or recent trauma.*

Question: What test should be done prior to administering heparin or thrombolytics?
Answer: *Stool hemoccult and coagulant studies.*

Question: What is the antidote for heparin?
Answer: *Protamine sulfate.*

Question: A patient allergic to fish might also be allergic to what medication?
Answer: *Protamine sulfate. It is derived from salmon sperm.*

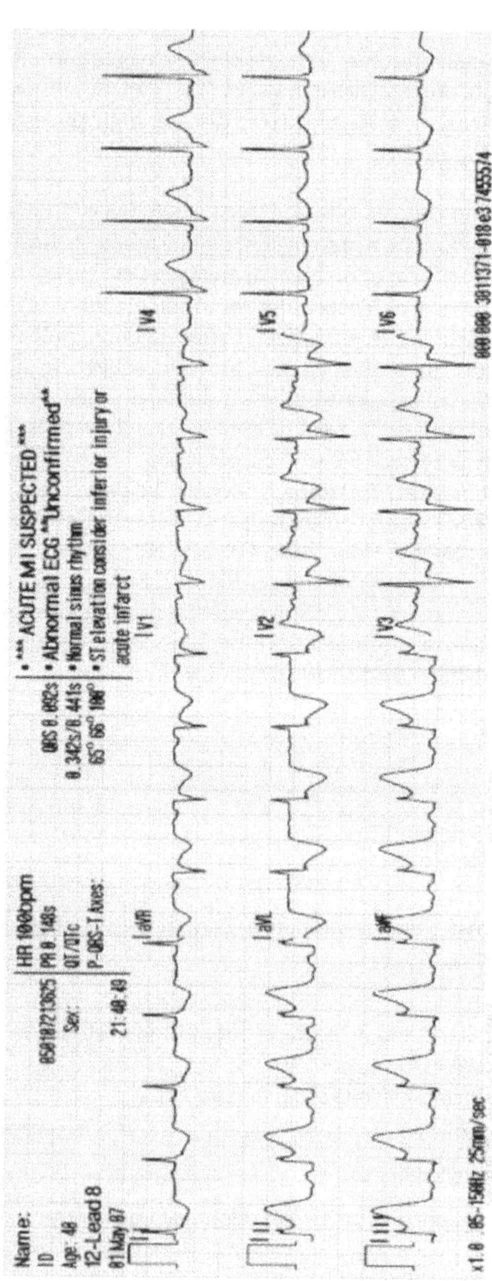

Figure 3.1 Suspected acute myocardial infarction.

ARTERIAL OCCLUSION

Arterial occlusion means a clogged artery.

- *Causes:* Coronary artery disease; atherosclerosis; hypertension; smoking; and hyperlipidemia.
- *Signs and symptoms:* Cool/pale extremities and weak pulse to the affected extremity.
- *Interventions:* Maintain extremity in **dependent position**; assess pulses through Doppler ultrasound; and prepare for possible surgery.

Notes: ____

____

____

____

____

____

____

____

____

____

____

____

____

____

____

____

____

ENDOCARDITIS

Endocarditis is an infection of the inner lining of the heart and/or the heart valves.

- *Causes:* Endocarditis occurs when a person with faulty heart valves contracts a common bacterial infection. For example, a bacterial infection in the skin can travel through the blood and attach to the faulty heart valve, resulting in endocarditis.
- *Signs and symptoms:* **P**etechiae, **S**hortness of breath, **F**ever and chills, **R**oth's spots, **O**sler's nodes, systolic **M**urmur, **J**aneway lesions (red spots on soles of feet), **A**nemia, **N**ail bed splinter hemorrhaging; **E**mboli, and chest pain. To remember these symptoms, just remember "**PS: FROM JANE.**"
- *Interventions:* Anticipate orders to obtain multiple blood cultures from multiple sites, administer antibiotics intravenously, and do a complete blood count.

Notes: ____

____

____

____

____

____

____

____

____

____

____

____

____

____

____

AORTIC INJURIES

Aortic injuries may occur anywhere on the ascending aorta, aortic arch, descending thoracic aorta, or abdominal aorta. The injuries can result in aneurysm, tear, or rupture. Without immediate surgery, the patient can bleed to death rapidly. So it is critical for the nurse to identify an aortic injury early.

- *Causes:* A history of aortic injuries may reveal hypertension; coronary artery disease; congestive heart failure; or a recent chest/abdominal trauma.
- *Signs and symptoms* (may vary depending on location): Hypotension; loss of consciousness; hypertension in upper extremities; stronger pulse in arms than in legs; **tearing chest pain** that radiates to the back; tearing abdominal pain; chest wall ecchymosis; and paraplegia.
- *Interventions:* Get patient on a stretcher; obtain vital signs; check blood pressure in all extremities; notify provider of patient signs and symptoms immediately; prepare for immediate surgery; start two large-bore IV lines; monitor cardiac performance; provide oxygen; perform EKG; and measure pulse oximetry.

Notes: ____

____

____

____

____

____

____

____

____

Question: Which type of trauma most commonly causes a descending thoracic aortic laceration?

Answer: *Deceleration trauma that causes shearing.*

SYMPTOMATIC BRADYCARDIA

In symptomatic bradycardia, heart rate is <60 beats per minute resulting in inadequate blood circulation. The patient is symptomatic, displaying signs of poor cardiac perfusion (see Figure 3.2).

- *Causes:* The cause is not always known, but underlying conditions such as coronary artery disease, heart disease, second- or third-degree heart blocks, hypertension, thyroid disease, medication overdose, and lung disease can contribute to bradycardia.
- *Signs and symptoms:* Heart rate <60 beats per minute; patient looks and feels unwell (e.g., altered loss of consciousness, chest pain, diaphoretic, and pale).
- *Interventions:* Assess airway, breathing, and circulation (ABCs); provide oxygen; check vital signs; measure pulse oxygen; perform EKG; monitor cardiac performance; anticipate orders to intravenously push 1.0 mg of atropine at 3- to 5-minute intervals, establish transcutaneous pacing, administer medications (dopamine or epinephrine), and prepare for transcutaneous (external) or internal pacer.

Notes: ____

____

____

____

____

____

____

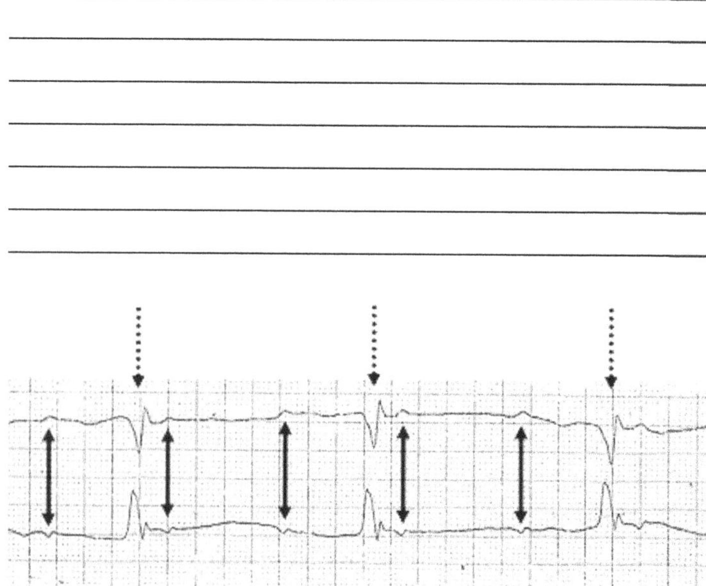

Figure 3.2 Symptomatic bradycardia.

SUPRAVENTRICULAR TACHYCARDIA

In supraventricular tachycardia, the heart rate is regular with **narrow complexes**, but it beats at >150 beats per minute. Supraventricular tachycardia can be divided into symptomatic/unstable (patient looks unwell) or asymptomatic/stable (patient looks fine; see Figure 3.3).

- *Causes:* The cause is not always known. However, some habits and conditions can contribute to it, such as stress, caffeine, smoking, cocaine use, alcohol use, thyroid disease, heart failure, pulmonary embolism, chronic obstructive pulmonary disease, and pneumonia. Some medications for asthma, cold medications, and digoxin can also contribute to supraventricular tachycardia.
- *Signs and symptoms:* Palpitations; chest pain; diaphoresis; anxiety; and pulse rate >150 beats per minute.
- *Interventions:*
  - *If patient is symptomatic and unstable,* anticipate order to prepare for immediate synchronized cardioversion 50 to 100 J biphasic.
  - *If patient is asymptomatic and stable,* anticipate orders to attempt vasovagal maneuvers, monitor cardiac performance, open large-bore IV line, provide oxygen, check vital signs, measure pulse oxygen, perform EKG, administer adenosine rapidly by IV push, and slow down atrioventricular (AV) conduction with beta-blockers/calcium channel blockers/ digoxin or amiodarone.
  - Give patient a coffee straw and ask the patient to blow through it to assist vagal maneuvers.

Notes: ____

____

____

____

____

____

____

____

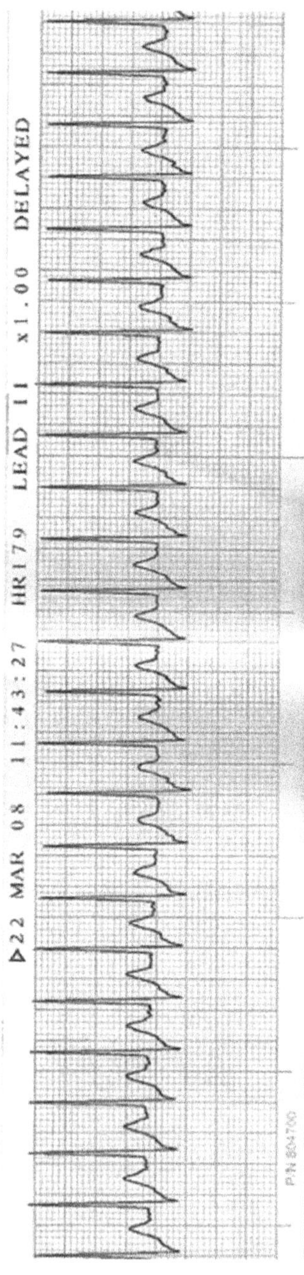

Figure 3.3 Supraventricular tachycardia.

VENTRICULAR FIBRILLATION OR PULSELESS VENTRICULAR TACHYCARDIA

Ventricular fibrillation (VF) and pulseless ventricular tachycardia (VT) are both irregular rapid rhythms in which there is no pulse (see Figure 3.4 and Table 3.1).

- *Causes:* Poor cardiac perfusion due to coronary artery disease; shock; hypokalemia; myocardial infarct; or electrocution.
- *Signs and symptoms:* Decreased level of consciousness; no pulse; VF or VT on cardiac monitor.
- *Interventions:* Assess for a pulse within 10 seconds; if no pulse present, call for help while initiating CPR starting with chest compressions; do not interrupt chest compressions while applying cardiac monitor/defibrillation pads. Pulseless VT or VF are shockable rhythms. Be sure you know how to set your machine to defibrillation mode and always make sure your team is all clear before pressing the shock button. Anticipate orders to administer early defibrillation, early epinephrine, and amiodarone or lidocaine per advanced cardiovascular life support protocols. Just remember **DEAL: D**efibrillation, **E**pinephrine, and **A**miodarone or **L**idocaine.

Notes: ____

Table 3.1

Pulseless Ventricular Tachycardia or Ventricular Fibrillation Treatment

1. Shock at 120–200 J biphasic
   - CPR 30/2 for five cycles or 2 min
   - Establish IV or IO access and administer epinephrine 1 mg IV/IO during CPR every 3–5 minutes

2. Shock at 200 J biphasic if still pulseless VT or VF after 2 min CPR
   - CPR 30/2 for five cycles or 2 min
   - Amiodarone 300 mg, 150 mg second dose, or lidocaine during CPR

3. Shock at 200 J biphasic if still pulseless VT or VF after 2 min CPR
   - CPR 30/2 for five cycles or 2 min
   - Consider magnesium 1–2 g IV/IO for torsades de pointes

IO, intraosseous; IV, intravenous; VF, ventricular fibrillation; VT, ventricular tachycardia.

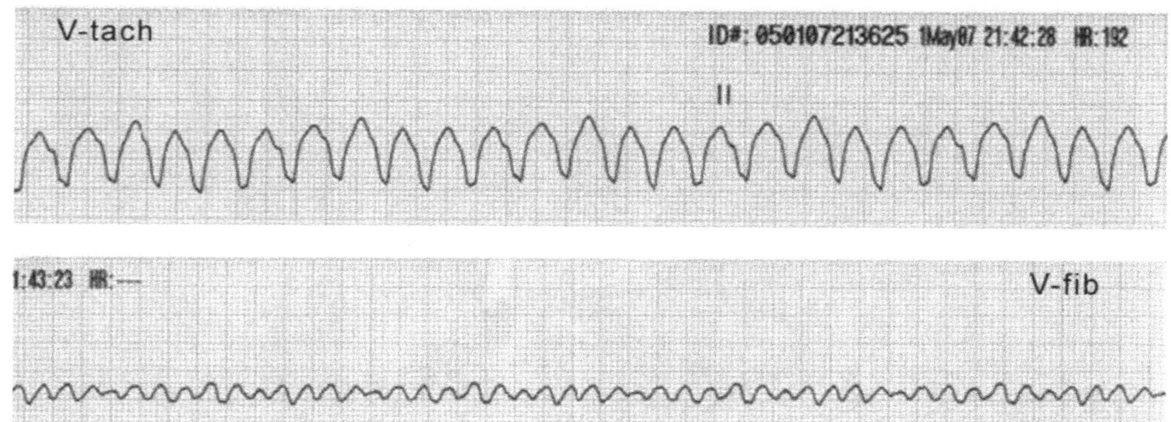

Figure 3.4 Ventricular fibrillation.

Question: If none of the previously mentioned interventions work, what are some other causes of VF?

Answer: *Hypothermia, hypoxia, hypoglycemia, overdose, cardiac tamponade, tension pneumothorax, trauma, acidosis, hypovolemia, and electrolyte imbalances.*

Question: You see VF on the monitor, but your patient is asymptomatic, sitting up, and talking to you. What is your first intervention?

Answer: *Check for a pulse. You cannot believe everything you see on a monitor; it could be artifact.*

Question: What is the maximum number of times one can safely defibrillate a patient?

Answer: *There is no limit.*

Question: Why do we defibrillate?

Answer: *To temporarily produce asystole. This may sound incorrect, but defibrillation actually depolarizes the heart, allowing the natural pacemakers of the heart to kick in.*

Question: What dose of lidocaine should be administered to patients with renal failure or liver failure, or patients who are older adults?

Answer: *Give half doses of lidocaine to patients with renal failure, patients with liver failure, or patients who are older adults.*

PULSELESS ELECTRICAL ACTIVITY

Pulseless electrical activity occurs when a rhythm shows on the monitor, but the patient does not have a pulse. Again, you cannot always believe what you see on the monitor.

- *Causes:* Can be attributed to the five Hs or five Ts.
    - Hypovolemia, Hypoxia, Hydrogen ion (acidosis), **Hyper-/hypokalemia**, or **Hypothermia**.
    - Toxin (drug overdose), Tamponade/cardiac, Tension pneumothorax, Thrombosis, and Trauma.
- *Signs and symptoms:* Your patient has no pulse, but there is a rhythm on the monitor. Remember that just because there is electrical activity in the heart does not mean the heart is actually pumping.
- *Interventions:* Check for a pulse; if no pulse, perform CPR starting with chest compressions; per order, insert an IV line, monitor oxygen, and administer epinephrine. Consider naloxone (Narcan) for opioid overdose and treat the underlying causes.

Notes: ____

____

____

____

____

____

____

____

____

____

____

____

____

____

POST CARDIAC ARREST

You got them back from the grips of death, so now what do you do? The battle is over, but the war has just begun. Your unstable patient is not really out of the woods so to speak; achieving stability will require a great team effort.

- *Causes:* Return of spontaneous circulation after cardiopulmonary arrest.
- *Signs and symptoms:* The patient will have regained a pulse after CPR. In most cases, the patient will remain unresponsive, hypotensive, and in need of respiratory and/or circulatory support.
- *Interventions:* Document a full primary assessment (ABCs + neurologic). Treat any known underlying causes of cardiopulmonary arrest. Assist A&E provider with establishment definitive airway (intubation and ventilator) as needed. Maintain pulse oxygenation between 92% and 98% and monitor capnography. Document Glasgow Coma Scale (GCS), pupillary, and complete neurologic assessment. Anticipate provider insertion of central IV line with central venous pressure (CVP) monitoring if available. Anticipate diagnostic test such as ABG, complete blood count (CBC), complete metabolic panel (CMP), Mg, phosphorus, calcium, prothrombin time (PT)/international normalized ratio (INR), partial thromboplastin time (PTT), lactate, creatine kinase MB (CK-MB), troponin, amylase, lipase, beta human chorionic gonadotropin (hCG) on childbearing women without prior hysterectomy, blood glucose, 12-lead EKG, portable chest X-ray (CXR), and head CT scan. **To preserve organs and prevent fever, consider targeted temperature management (TTM).** Evaluate if patient meets TTM criteria per hospital protocol such as
    - GCS score below 9 to 6 per hospital policy,
    - Remaining unresponsive continually for 15 to 30 minutes post cardiac arrest,
    - Receiving CPR for <45 minutes, and
    - NO signs of bleeding or coagulopathies as **hypothermia increases bleeding.**

If patient meets TTM criteria, **obtain head CT prior to attaching the cooling unit to the patient to check for cerebral hemorrhage.** Insert core temperature monitoring device (esophageal and/or Foley temperature-sensing probes are more effective than rectal). Attach the cooling unit to the patient according to the manufacture guidelines. **Goal-targeted core temperature will be 33 °C to 36 °C per order.** Typically, patients with cerebral edema will require lower 33 °C, otherwise 36 °C can be just as effective. Goal time for initiation of TTM is within **4 hours** per policy. Anticipate orders to administer sedatives and paralytics to prevent shivering. Monitor for anticipated bradycardia, hypotension, hypokalemia, and hypoglycemia during TTM. Prepare for ICU admission where rewarming phase will occur very gradually over about 24 to 36 hours.

Question: What is the effect of nitroprusside (Nipride) administered intravenously?
Answer: *It reduces afterload and increases cardiac output. It decreases myocardial oxygen demand without affecting the heart rate.*

Question: What type of EKG changes might you see in a patient with a potassium level of 7.8?
Answer: *Bradycardia, peaked T waves, and widened QRS complex.*

Question: What equation defines cardiac output?
Answer: *Heart rate × stroke volume.*

Question: What are the manifestations of digoxin toxicity?
Answer: *Blurred vision, halos, and arrhythmias.*

Question: What is the treatment for digoxin toxicity?
Answer: *Glucagon, phenytoin (Dilantin), and digoxin immune fab (Digibind).*

Question: Name three vasopressors.
Answer: *Norepinephrine, dopamine, and metaraminol are vasopressors.*

Question: What is the antidote for warfarin (Coumadin)?
Answer: *Vitamin K.*

Essential Facts

- Heparin affects partial thromboplastin time.
- Warfarin (Coumadin) affects prothrombin time.
- Pro tip: Amiodarone can precipitate when diluted. When hanging an amiodarone drip, be sure to attach an in-line filter to prevent phlebitis. Also check your rate as the dose tapers down after the first 6 hours.

SUMMARY

Although cardiovascular diseases threaten lives every day, they can often be resolved with quick treatment. Make EKG a priority for all patients with chest pain. **Arrival to EKG should be <7 minutes per hospital protocol**. Study and understand the various dysrhythmias and their treatments. Print out a rhythm strip on your monitored patients and add it to the patient's chart per shift and as needed. An A&E nurse needs to understand the basics of cardiovascular assessments and treatments and be certified in advanced cardiovascular life support.

4

Dental, Ear, Nose, and Throat Emergencies

Dental, ear, nose, and throat emergencies are daily occurrences in the A&E. Most of the time, they are not life threatening. From **foreign objects to trauma or infection**, this chapter takes you through the most common dental, ear, nose, and throat emergencies you will face. Be sure to practice using the otoscope and ophthalmic scope and document your assessment findings. Upon completing this chapter, you will be able to differentiate between the nonurgent and emergent dental, ear, nose, and throat emergencies. For each emergency, you will learn causes, manifestations, and interventions.

During this part of your orientation, locate and become familiar with:

- Dental repair kit and its contents
- Alligator forceps
- Ear wicks
- Eardrops for infection and cerumen impaction
- Ear irrigation supplies and ear curettes
- Headlamp and otoscope

DENTAL ABSCESS

A dental abscess is a pocket of infection and/or pus located in the gums near the base of a tooth.

- *Causes:*
  - *Periodontal abscess:* An infection of the soft tissue related to periodontitis (gum disease) or foreign object.
  - *Periapical abscess:* An infection of the supporting bone around the root structure caused by damage to the pulp (nerve and blood supply) of the tooth.
- *Signs and symptoms:* Manifestation may vary depending on location but usually includes pain, swelling, toothache, tenderness, fever, and foul breath. Infection may be localized but may also spread into areas of the face and neck. Pain may radiate to neck, jaw, and ear.
- *Interventions:* Assess and treat any airway obstructions first. Anticipate orders to set up oral anesthetics and incision and drainage tray or supplies, and administer any intravenous fluids, pain medication, and antibiotics as ordered. Anticipate diagnostic study orders such as complete blood count, arterial blood gas, erythrocyte sedimentation rate, wound cultures of the abscess, and CT or soft-tissue x-ray of the head and neck. Instruct the patient to take prescriptions as ordered, rinse with warm salt water, and **follow up with a dentist.**

Notes: ____

FRACTURED TOOTH

A tooth fracture is a broken or chipped tooth. This commonly occurs to the "two front teeth" or anterior maxillary teeth related to facial trauma.

- *Causes:* Oral, facial, or head trauma.
- *Signs and symptoms:* Vary according to type and location of trauma and may include broken or chipped tooth, bleeding at site of injury, pain, swelling, and/or embedded tooth fragments.

- *Interventions:* If facial trauma is present, stabilize any airway, breathing, or circulation concerns first. Consider tooth aspiration. Then place warm, moist cotton over the exposed tooth fracture and cover with dry gauze. Administer oral analgesics and tetanus vaccine as ordered. Consider abuse if caregiver history does not match that of the patient. Referral to a dentist within 24 to 48 hours of injury is critical for proper tooth repair. Set up emergency dental repair kit for provider administration.

Notes: ____

Essential Facts

An emergency dental repair kit, box, or supplies for provider administration may include zinc oxide, nerve-blocking agent, calcium hydroxide, intermediate restorative material (IMR), dental foil, dental cement, and/or dry socket paste.

ODONTALGIA

"Odontalgia" is a big fancy word for dental caries or "cavities." Commonly, patients show up to the A&E for the severe pain associated with odontalgia.

- *Causes:* Poor oral hygiene and a diet high in sugar. Infants and children can acquire cavities if given a bottle to drink at bedtime.
- *Signs and symptoms:* Pain; gray or blackened area noted on affected tooth; toothache; and neck or facial swelling.
- *Interventions:* May include administration of topical anesthetics, nerve blocks, narcotic analgesics, IMR, and antibiotics. However, these treatments do not cure odontalgia; they simply buy the patient some time until the patient sees the dentist. Stress the importance of good oral hygiene and need for following up with the dentist during discharge instructions.

Notes: ____

TOOTH AVULSION

Tooth avulsion occurs when the whole tooth is removed from its socket. This is a time-sensitive emergency. The best chance of saving the tooth is reimplantation *within 20 to 30 minutes.*

- *Causes:* Commonly head, facial, or oral trauma of some sort.
- *Signs and symptoms:* Missing tooth; bleeding; pain; and swelling. Hopefully, your patient found the missing tooth and brought it in to the A&E with them.
- *Interventions:* If facial trauma is present, stabilize any airway, breathing, or circulation concerns first. Consider tooth aspiration. Tooth and socket should be gently cleansed with tap water or saline and any debris removed. Attempt should be made to place the cleansed tooth back in its socket. If tooth will not stay in socket, tooth should be placed in a liquid medium such as milk or saliva. Administer oral analgesics and tetanus vaccine as ordered. Referral to a dentist within 24 to 48 hours of injury is critical for proper tooth repair. Set up dental repair kit, box, or supplies for provider administration as ordered. Discharge teaching should include the use of helmets and mouth guards when playing sports.

Notes: ____

Question: Which liquid media are appropriate for avulsed teeth?
Answer: *Saliva, milk, saline, or Hank's solution (an over-the-counter product).*

LUDWIG'S ANGINA

Ludwig's angina occurs when a preexisting dental infection or cellulitis spreads into the sublingual, submandibular, and/or submental mandibular spaces.

- *Causes:* The spreading of a preexisting dental infection.
- *Signs and symptoms:* Anterior or lateral neck swelling; tongue swelling; muffled voice; pain; drooling; dysphagia; fever; and chills.
- *Interventions:* The swelling related to this particular type of infection places your patient at **high risk for airway obstruction.**

Assess and maintain patent airway, breathing, and circulation. Anticipate orders to administer oxygen, intravenous fluids, pain medication, and antibiotics; attach pulse oximeter and cardiac monitor; set up for incision and drainage; and/or prepare for operating room (OR) admission. Diagnostic tests may include arterial blood gas, complete blood count, erythrocyte sedimentation rate, culture of oral infected wound or drainage, and head and neck soft-tissue x-rays or CT.

Notes: ____

EAR EMERGENCIES

FOREIGN OBJECTS

You name it, and it can be found in an ear or a nostril. It commonly occurs with curious young children and toddlers but occasionally with adult patients. Hopefully, the object will be detected before infection occurs. Getting it out of the uncooperative 3-year-old patient is the real trick!

- *Causes:* Foreign object in the ear, such as nuts, bolts, raisins, peas, beads, bugs, and cotton.
- *Signs and symptoms:* Visible foreign object; purulent or bloody discharge; discomfort or pain; swelling; redness; foul odor; and foreign body sensation.
- *Interventions:*
  - Assist A&E provider in removing the foreign body with suction, irrigation, alligator forceps, ear curette, or even the pacer magnet for metal objects. Caution should be taken to avoid further dislodging it deeper into the nose or ear and possible aspiration with nasal foreign bodies. Provide ear antibiotics or nasal decongestants as ordered. Instruct the patient not to put anything smaller than an elbow in their ears or nose!
  - Sometimes, nasal foreign bodies can be dislodged simply by closing off the unaffected nostril and asking the patient to blow forcefully out of the affected nostril.
  - If unable to remove foreign body, provider may refer patient to ear, nose, and throat specialist.

Notes: ____

CERUMEN IMPACTION

- *Causes:* Buildup of ear wax that blocks the ear drum. Use of cotton swabs deep inside the ear canal can push wax deeper into the ear canal leading to wax impaction.
- *Signs and symptoms:* Asymptomatic or muffled/decreased hearing, earache, tinnitus, and dizziness.

There are many ways to flush an ear, but this seems to work the best for wax removal.

- First, gather lukewarm water with a splash of peroxide mixed in a small basin and a 20-mL syringe with plastic needle-less short tip. To make a needle-less plastic tip, you can also cut the plastic end of an intravenous catheter to measure approximately 1 cm in length.
- Lay the patient on their side with affected ear up. Fill the ear canal with warm water and peroxide solution and let soak for 10 minutes. You can use that 10 minutes to get some charting done, update vital signs, or complete your assessment. Then sit patient up with basin under ear to catch fluids. Now that the wax is softened, irrigate ear canal using syringe with plastic needle-less tip and rest of water solution. If a brown scaly pebble comes out, this is the wax impaction; you got it!

Notes: ____

ACUTE OTITIS EXTERNA (SWIMMER'S EAR)

Acute otitis externa is a bacterial or fungal infection of the outer ear.

- *Causes:* Outer ear infections commonly occur because of frequent swimming or foreign objects in the ear. Bacteria or fungus enters with the water or the foreign object, thereby causing an infection.
- *Signs and symptoms:* Outer ear pain; itchy, impaired hearing; ear discharge; fever; erythema; and swelling of the outer ear.
- *Interventions:* Give topical eardrop solution/antibiotics as ordered; provide ear wick; and use warm compresses. Instruct the patient not to swim until the infection is resolved (7–10 days).

Notes: ____

When examining the ear in an adult, pull *up* and back; in a child under 3 years of age, pull the ear *down* and back.

ACUTE OTITIS MEDIA

Acute otitis media is a middle-ear bacterial or viral infection. It is more common in children because of their short, narrow Eustachian tubes. An infant or toddler with otitis media may appear irritable; cry; pull at ears; and have a poor appetite, nausea, vomiting, or diarrhea.

- *Causes:* Middle-ear infections usually start as a sinus infection.
- *Signs and symptoms:* Recent upper respiratory infection; earache; impaired hearing; red or dull gray bulging tympanic membrane; and fever.
- *Interventions:* Administer and evaluate effectiveness of antipyretics, antibiotics, and pain medication as ordered.

Notes: ____

ACUTE OTITIS INTERNA (LABYRINTHITIS)

An inflammation to the labyrinth part of the inner ear, which control balance and hearing. Typically affects adults.

- *Causes:* Viral or bacterial infection.
- *Signs and symptoms:* Loss of hearing, nausea, vomiting, tinnitus, imbalance, and **severe vertigo.**
- *Interventions:* Meclizine, antiemetics, antihistamines, antibiotics if bacterial infection, bed rest, driving restrictions.

Notes: ____

RUPTURED TYMPANIC MEMBRANE

This is a tear or rupture of the tympanic membrane (eardrum).

- *Causes:* Tears may be the result of **bacterial infection** or trauma from a foreign object (Q-tip, bobby pin) or other forces (e.g., explosions, skull fractures, burns).

- *Signs and symptoms:* Ear pain; discharge; impaired hearing; vertigo; nausea, vomiting, and fever.
- *Interventions:* With most small perforations, the eardrum grows back on its own, similar to the way a fingernail grows back. Anticipate orders to administer oral antibiotics, prepare for surgery in large perforations; instruct patient not to blow nose or get ears wet, and provide follow-up with an ear, nose, and throat specialist.

Notes: ____

MÉNIÈRE'S DISEASE

Ménière's disease is a long-term progressive inner-ear disorder affecting approximately 1 out of every 1,000 to 2,000 people.

- *Causes:* Its cause is unknown but has been linked to abnormal amounts of fluid in the inner ear. Symptoms usually occur suddenly and can last from a few minutes to a few hours.
- *Signs and symptoms:* **Vertigo**; dizziness; nausea and vomiting; tinnitus; impaired hearing; diaphoresis; headache; balancing difficulties; and blurred vision.
- *Interventions:* Bring side rails up (fall precautions) and put the bed in the low-locked position; speak slowly and clearly; administer meclizine or diazepam (intravenously) for rapid relief and antiemetics as ordered; require bed rest and a quiet environment; and provide diet instructions (low sodium, no caffeine, and no nicotine).

Notes: ____

NASAL EMERGENCIES

ALLERGIC RHINITIS (HAY FEVER)

Rhinitis is a nasal mucous membrane inflammation.

- *Causes:* Allergic response to pollen, dust, or other allergens. It may be acute (seasonal) or chronic (perennial).
- *Signs and symptoms:* Watery nasal drainage; nasal congestion; sneezing; cough; and sore throat. Infants may present with difficulty breathing or poor feeding.

- *Interventions:* Administer medications as ordered (analgesics, antibiotics, decongestants, and antihistamines); increase fluid intake; and perform bulb syringe suction in infants.

Notes: ____

EPISTAXIS

Epistaxis is a nosebleed. There are two types: anterior bleeds and posterior bleeds.

Anterior bleeds are more common and easier to control.

- *Causes:* Trauma; cocaine use; disease; nose picking; or just dry air during winter months.
- *Signs and symptoms:* Bright red nasal bleeding.
- *Interventions:* Position patient sitting up and leaning forward; apply direct pressure to bridge of nose; apply ice; administer medications as ordered (topical tranexamic acid or pseudoephedrine); and prepare for cauterization or nasal packing.

Posterior bleeds are less common and more difficult to control.

- *Causes:* Usually associated with chronic medical problems, such as hypertension, blood dyscrasia, or tumor.
- *Signs and symptoms:* Nasal bleeding.
- *Interventions:* Apply direct pressure and ice for 10 minutes or more. Position the patient sitting up and leaning forward over a large basin. Establish large-bore intravenous access, if ordered; have suction and headlamp available; arrange for ear, nose, and throat consult as ordered; prepare for procedure (posterior nasal packing, nasal tampon, or cauterization); and monitor level of consciousness, vital signs, pulse oxygen, and bleeding. *Instruct patient not to blow nose.*

Notes: ____

NASAL FRACTURE

This is a fracture of the nasal bones.

- *Causes:* Direct trauma to the nose.
- *Signs and symptoms:* Nasal bleeding; nasal ecchymosis or edema; nasal airway obstruction; and deformity or tenderness over nasal bridge.

- *Interventions:* Control bleeding with direct pressure; apply ice; administer analgesics as ordered and evaluate effectiveness; and arrange for nasal or facial x-ray. *Instruct patient not to blow nose.*
  - If nasal airway is not obstructed, no treatment is necessary.
  - If nasal airway is obstructed, patient will be referred to an ear, nose, and throat specialist for repair *1 week after swelling decreases.*

Notes: ____

SINUSITIS

Sinusitis is a sinus inflammation.

- *Causes:* Infection; allergies; chemical irritants; pressure changes; cocaine use; dental abscesses; or mechanical obstruction.
- *Signs and symptoms:* Pain; purulent nasal drainage; and fever.
- *Interventions:* Anticipate orders to administer medications and evaluate effectiveness (decongestants, antibiotic, and analgesic/ narcotic); and arrange for sinus films or CT scan.

Notes: ____

THROAT EMERGENCIES

PHARYNGITIS/TONSILLITIS

This is inflammation of the throat or tonsils.

- *Causes:* Bacterial or viral infection.
- *Signs and symptoms:* Sore throat; red, swollen tonsils; white pus on tonsils; difficulty swallowing; fever; ear pain; foul breath; and swollen cervical lymph nodes.
- *Interventions:* Arrange for strep or monospot test; administer antibiotic by mouth (PO) or intramuscular (IM) injection as ordered; and monitor airway patency.
  - Soft-tissue neck x-ray may be used to rule out *epiglottitis* or retropharyngeal abscess when patient demonstrates pain, drooling, "hot-potato voice," or difficulty in breathing.

Notes: ____

PERITONSILLAR ABSCESS

This is an abscess of the tonsil. It may be a respiratory emergency if the airway is obstructed.

- *Causes:* Commonly caused by streptococcus bacteria.
- *Signs and symptoms:* Sore throat; **unilateral swollen tonsil**; swollen cervical lymph nodes; dysphagia; fever; difficulty in opening mouth; swollen palate; laterally displaced uvula; **drooling**; and muffled or "hot-potato voice."
- *Interventions:* Prepare for incision and drainage of abscess with ear, nose, and throat consultant; administer antibiotics and pulse oxygen; and monitor airway.

Notes: ____

Question: What is the difference between tonsillitis and peritonsillar abscess?

Answer: *With tonsillitis, both tonsils are swollen. With peritonsillar abscess, one tonsil is swollen.*

SUMMARY

You should now have a basic understanding of the dental, ear, nose, and throat problems that are seen daily in the A&E. Do not be afraid to take an otoscope and assess your patient's mouth, gums, and teeth, ears, nose, or throat. Document your pre- and post-intervention findings. Most providers appreciate a good assessment, especially one that is well documented before and after treatment.

5

Disaster Response Emergencies

Working in the A&E automatically makes you a first responder during a local, national, or global disaster. Therefore, it is vital to know your role, communicate effectively, and locate equipment quickly. Disasters can be divided into two categories: natural and man made. This chapter opens with the definitions, categories, and interventions for disasters. Many nurses may find remembering disaster instructions difficult because, quite simply, they are rarely used. Never fear. Just learn these three helpful mnemonics to remember what to do: **DISASTER, SALT,** and **IDME.** Then, the chapter guides you through some of the most common radiologic, chemical, and biological exposures. Again, you may find it challenging to remember information that is used so infrequently, so just keep this book and the Centers for Disease Control and Prevention (CDC) website handy. These two sources will provide all the information you need. To fully understand the material and ease your anxiety, be sure to practice regular disaster drills in your facility. Pay attention to the methods of communication, disaster triage, and preparedness available in your hospital.

During this part of your orientation, locate and become familiar with:

- Your facility's disaster plans and incident command system
- Your facility's disaster codes
- Decontamination equipment
- Fire alarms and extinguishers
- Oxygen shut-off valves

- Evacuation plans and routes
- Disaster documentation
- Contacts/whom to notify if a disaster occurs
- Where to sign up to participate in a disaster drill
- Disaster alternative communication routes
- Personal protective equipment (PPE) for highly infectious diseases
- Hazmat suits
- Hospital disaster supplies and tags

TYPES OF DISASTERS

A "disaster" is an event in which needs exceed resources. **The goal during a disaster is to do the greatest good for the greatest number of people.** The types are indicated in Table 5.1.

Table 5.1

Types of Disasters

Natural	Man made
Hurricane	Explosion
Earthquake	Fire
Landslide	Firearms
Ice storm/blizzard	Stampede
Fire	Structural collapse
Wildfire	Hazardous material
Flood	Power out
Tidal wave	Blocked communications
Tornado	Transportation event:
Asteroid collision	■ Airway (plane)
	■ Railway (train)
Avalanche	■ Waterway (boat)
Volcanic eruption	■ Roadway (car)
Widespread highly contagious infections	Weapons of mass destruction:
	■ Biological
	■ Chemical
Epidemic or pandemic	■ Nuclear

INTERVENTIONS

To remember the proper interventions to follow in a disaster, remember the mnemonics DISASTER, SALT, and IDME.

Notes: ____

DISASTER

- *Detect:* What is the reason for the disaster? Are there mass casualties? Do our needs exceed our resources?
- *Incident command:* People trained to manage, coordinate, and organize the disaster operation. Do we need them and, if so, where?

Essential Facts

Homeland Security Presidential Directive 5 requires hospital staff to be trained on the incident command system.

- *Safe and secure scene:* This is the first step in disaster management. Is it safe? Always protect yourself and team members first, then the public, patients, and environment. Use **PPE, such as gown, gloves, mask,** and eye protection.
- *Assess hazards:* What are other potential hazards (e.g., downed power lines, chemicals, blood, smoke, leaking gas line, bad weather)?
- *Support:* What people and supplies are needed? Do we need hazmat team, fire and rescue team, law enforcement, vehicles, water? Do we need additional medical/nursing/support staff/ operating room (OR) teams, PPE, blood products, and water?
- *Triage and treatment:* Do we need disaster triage? How much treatment is required? Follow your facility's disaster triage plan. If your facility does not have one, you can locate one online through the Federal Emergency Management Agency (FEMA). See SALT and IDME mnemonics in the following.
- *Evacuate:* Can the victims be transported to a safe location and, if so, how?
- *Recovery:* What are some recovery issues?

Notes: ____

SALT

- *Sort* or prioritize patients into one of three categories based on movement by calling out to the victims:
  - "Those who can walk, come to this location." These are minimal Priority 3 (Green): able to walk.
  - "Those who can hear my voice, wave your hand." These are delayed Priority 2 (Yellow): able to wave with purposeful movement.
  - "Those who do not respond." These are immediate Priority 1 (Red): still with obvious threats to life.
- *Assess* the victims who cannot walk or move, as they are more urgent and need assistance.
- *Limited life-saving interventions:* If indicated, perform the following:
  - Open the airway through repositioning with jaw-thrust maneuver.
  - Perform needle chest decompression.
  - Control major hemorrhage with direct pressure or tourniquet.
  - Administer autoinjector antidotes.
- *Triage and transport:* Triage or sort patients using the IDME mnemonic. Transport the immediate first, then delayed, minimal, expectant, and dead.

Notes: ____

IDME

- *Immediate, Emergent, or Red acuity:* These victims have an alteration in airway, breathing, and circulation (ABCs) or threat to loss of life or limb.
- *Delayed, Urgent, or Yellow acuity:* These victims need medical attention, but they are not at risk of rapidly deteriorating.
- *Minimal, Nonurgent, or Green acuity (a.k.a. "The Walking Wounded"):* These victims have stable vital signs and minor wounds. Consider an alternative treatment location for these patients.
- *Expectant or Black acuity:* These victims have little or no chance of survival with current resources. Comfort measures should be given if available. Once all immediate and delayed patients have been treated, then available resources can be used on the expectant patients.

Send immediate victims to hospital/operating room/ICU first. Try to route these patients to a trauma center and divide the delayed patients between other facilities.

Notes: ____

Essential Facts

To remember the proper interventions to follow in a disaster, remember the mnemonics **DISASTER, SALT,** and **IDME.**

Never downgrade the initial disaster triage acuity to a less urgent acuity.

A mass casualty incident is not the same as a disaster. There is a sudden influx of patients that may be overwhelming but normal standards of care and protocols are used. During a disaster, normal standards of care are not possible.

Phases of Disaster

1. *Mitigation* is assessing potential disasters that may commonly occur in your area.
2. *Preparedness* is obtaining resources needed for potential disasters and practicing drills to determine other needs.
3. *Response* is responding to a disaster.
4. *Recovery* can take weeks to months or even years depending on the severity of the disaster.

RADIATION, CHEMICAL, AND BIOLOGICAL EXPOSURES

Be on the lookout for these in the event multiple patients come in with the same symptoms. Emergency medical personnel should **always wear PPE**, remove contaminated clothing, clean objects in 1% bleach solution, wash patient in proper decontamination showering systems, and **report to infection control at the CDC** at wwwn.cdc.gov/dcs/ContactUs/Form (1-800-CDC-INFO).

ABRIN OR RICIN TOXICITY

Abrin or ricin toxicity results from biological exposure to processed castor beans used to make castor oil.

- *Causes:* Contact with poison released from processed castor beans, such as might occur at a castor bean plant. The poison inactivates type II ribosomes in the body.
- *Signs and symptoms:* Within a few days, metabolic acidosis; hepatitis; renal failure; and hematuria.
  - *If poison is inhaled:* Within 4 to 8 hours, the patient will experience distress, fever, cough, shortness of breath, pulmonary edema, lung necrosis, and shock.

- *If poison is ingested:* Nausea, vomiting, and diarrhea; rectal bleeding; hypotension; gastrointestinal necrosis; and hepatitis.
- *Interventions:* Decontaminate the patient with proper equipment; use standard precautions; administer fluids intravenously per order; and avoid exposure to contaminated substances. There is no antidote; treat the symptoms. Charcoal may be ordered, if ingestion is recent.

Notes: ____

ANTHRAX

Anthrax is a spore-forming gram-positive bacteria (*Bacillus anthracis*).

- *Causes:* Contaminated soil, animals, and animal products. The bacteria enter the body through inhalation, skin, or ingestion.
- *Signs and symptoms:*
  - *If spore is inhaled:* Within 2 to 40+ days, flu-like symptoms, including weakness; cough; congestion; sore throat; fever; shortness of breath; respiratory distress; and shock occur.
  - *If spore enters subcutaneously:* Within a week, an itchy vesicle turns into an ulcer and then a black scab, possibly with fever (see Figure 5.1).
  - *If spore is ingested:* Within a week, nausea, vomiting, and diarrhea; rectal bleeding; and fever occur.
- *Interventions:* Anticipate orders to obtain blood cultures, arrange for chest x-ray and CT scan, give antibiotics such as ciprofloxacin, and use standard precautions. Antibiotics may not be effective against bacterial exotoxins increasing the mortality rate.

Notes: ____

Essential Facts

The inhaled form of anthrax has a very high fatality rate.

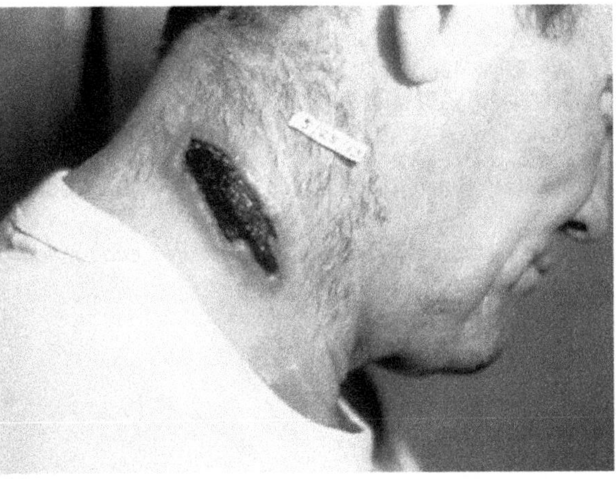

Figure 5.1 Subcutaneous anthrax.

BOTULISM

Botulism is a paralyzing exotoxin produced by the bacteria *Clostridium botulinum*.

- *Causes:* Contaminated food; infected wounds; and spore consumption (e.g., honey) by infants.
- *Signs and symptoms:* Within 4 days, patient has multiple cranial nerve palsies. The patient is also afebrile with bilateral facial droop; dysphonia; blurred vision; normal mental status; dry mouth; dysphagia; dysarthria; and bilateral descending skeletal muscle paralysis (opposite of Guillain-Barre which is ascending paralysis). Respiratory failure occurs in 24 hours or less.
- *Interventions:* Maintain standard precautions; assess neurologic status; monitor cardiac performance; measure pulse oxygen; collect gastric or stool samples; use ventilator if patient is experiencing respiratory failure; and give antitoxin available through state health departments and the CDC as ordered.

Notes: ____

Question: An infant is brought into the A&E for facial droop, muscle weakness, and shallow respirations. Botulism is suspected. What does this patient need from the CDC?
Answer: *Antitoxin.*

True or False: Botox contains minute amounts of botulinum to smooth wrinkles.
Answer: *True. 1 ounce (30 g) of pure exotoxin is enough to kill everyone in the United States.*

BLISTER AGENT (MUSTARD GAS)

A blister agent is an alkaline agent with a mustard, onion, or garlic odor.

- *Causes:* The gas is an agent used in chemical warfare that results in blisters and burns.
- *Signs and symptoms:* Within 12 hours, the patient experiences second-degree burns; skin redness with blisters; corneal abrasions; sore throat; nausea, vomiting, and diarrhea; cough; and difficulty in breathing.
- *Interventions:* Decontaminate patient; assess ABCs first; and treat symptoms, particularly chemical burns, with topical antibiotics as ordered. There is no antidote.

Notes: ____

BRUCELLOSIS

Brucellosis is a bacterial (*Brucella*) infection.

- *Causes:* Infected animals or animal products.
- *Signs and symptoms:* Within 4 weeks, the patient experiences fever; flu-like symptoms; sweating; headache; weakness; hepatitis; joint pain; arthritis; osteomyelitis; and endocarditis.
- *Interventions:* Use standard precautions; and anticipate orders to obtain blood cultures and give antibiotics (doxycycline and rifampin).

Notes: ____

CYANIDE

Cyanide is a colorless chemical gas or crystal that binds with cellular mitochondria preventing adenosine triphosphate (ATP) production. It has a bitter almond odor. Example: the "Jonestown Massacre" of 1978, where 909 Americans died by drinking cyanide-poisoned punch or Kool-Aid.

- *Causes:* Gas or crystals found in manufacturing; certain foods; smoke inhalation; and cigarette smoke. Fire can cause cyanide to be released from plastic, wool, silk, cotton, foam, synthetic rubber, and other synthetic products. A house fire survivor with smoke inhalation may also have cyanide poisoning.
- *Signs and symptoms:* Bradypnea; dizziness; weakness; headache; nausea; vomiting; tachycardia or bradycardia; hypotension; loss of consciousness; and respiratory failure.
- *Interventions:* Decontaminate patient; assess and treat ABCs; and give cyanide antidote as ordered.

Notes: ____

NERVE AGENTS

Nerve agents are chemical agents that block nerve impulses causing paralysis. Example: Sarin gas in 1995 Tokyo subway attack.

- *Causes:* These agents can be absorbed through the skin or inhaled and block neuromuscular junction enzymes.
- *Signs and symptoms:* Remember **SLUDGE** (Saliva, Lacrimation, Urination, Defecation, GI upset, and Emesis—everything is wet). Early symptoms include tachycardia; lethargy; paralysis; shock; anxiety; bronchospasms; ataxia; and pulmonary edema.
- *Interventions:* Decontaminate the patient. If the agent was ingested orally, anticipate orders to give 1 g/kg of charcoal. Other orders may include atropine to reverse central nervous system effects; Atrovent (ipratropium) nebulizer to dry secretions; pralidoxime (2-PAM) slowly over 30 minutes or obidoxime.

Notes: ____

PLAGUE

Plague is a contagious bacterial infection (*Yersinia pestis*). Example: "Black Death" or "Great Plague" of the 14th century killed millions in Asia, Africa, and Europe.

- *Causes:* This bacterial infection is found endemically in animals. It spreads directly by infected flea bites to humans and other animals. Its three types are bubonic, septicemic, and pneumonic.
- *Signs and symptoms (see Figure 5.2):*
  - *Bubonic:* Within 1 week, acute fever; chills; weakness; painful, swollen lymph nodes (buboes).
  - *Septicemic:* Fever; chills; weakness; blackened necrotic extremities; abdominal pain; and sepsis.
  - *Pneumonic:* Fever; headache; weakness; dyspnea; hemoptysis; chest pain; rapid and severe pneumonia; respiratory failure; and shock. It is the only type that can be spread via droplets.
- *Interventions:* Droplet precautions. Anticipate orders to obtain intravenous (IV) access; arrange for chest x-ray; arrange lymph node aspiration; collect blood and sputum cultures; and give antibiotics (streptomycin or gentamicin).

Notes: ____

Question: How is the plague most commonly transmitted to humans?

Answer: *By* direct *contact with infected rodent fleas.*

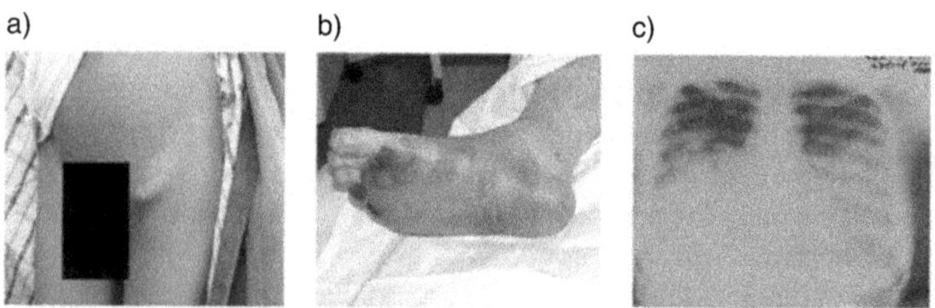

a) b) c)

Figure 5.2 Forms of plague: (a) bubonic plague, (b) septicemic plague, and (c) pneumonic plague.
Source: www.cdc.gov/plague/symptoms/index.html

Q-FEVER

Q-fever is a *Coxiella burnetii* bacterial infection. Complications may include hepatitis, myocarditis, and pneumonia.

- *Causes: Coxiella burnetii* bacteria found in animals and animal products (**unpasteurized milk**).
- *Signs and symptoms:* Within 2 to 3 weeks, the patient experiences flu-like symptoms (high fevers; cough; fatigue; nausea, vomiting, and diarrhea); abdominal pain; and chest pain.
- *Interventions:* Maintain standard precautions; anticipate orders to obtain complete blood count, liver enzymes, metabolic panel, chest x-ray, and cultures; and give antibiotics (doxycycline and ciprofloxacin).

Notes: ____

CORONAVIRUSES

Coronaviruses are a zoonotic family of viruses that can infect humans or animals and have resulted in previous epidemics and pandemics. Middle Eastern Respiratory Syndrome (MERS), Severe Acute Respiratory Syndrome (SARS), and coronavirus disease 2019 (COVID-19) are examples of coronaviruses.

- *Causes:* Coronaviruses are believed to be of animal origin, possibly bats and dromedary camels. It is possible that the asymptomatic or undetected cases may lead to the rapid spread of coronaviruses.
- *Signs and symptoms:* Symptoms may vary in severity ranging from asymptomatic to mild cases, which resemble a cold, to severe cases, which result in acute respiratory distress syndrome (ARDS). These symptoms include headache, fatigue, body aches, dry cough, fever, congestion, sore throat, loss of taste or smell, nausea, vomiting, diarrhea, difficulty in breathing, pneumonia, pulmonary edema, septic shock, respiratory distress, and/or respiratory failure.
- *Interventions:* Identify possibility of coronavirus infection using triage and travel screening. Then initiate airborne droplet and contact-isolation precautions per facility protocol. Inform infectious disease personnel. Treatment is supportive. Prophylactic COVID-19 vaccines are recommended. Routine aerosolized respiratory treatments and procedures may be avoided or restricted to reduce spreading the virus in the air. Full airborne droplet precautions may be required including eye protection, N95

mask or procedure mask, gown, and gloves. **Epidemic or pandemic spread of coronaviruses can rapidly deplete resources and strain the healthcare systems.** Consider plans to conserve PPE and sanitizing materials. Document a thorough respiratory assessment. Anticipate orders to obtain coronavirus nasopharyngeal sample, chest x-ray, IV access, blood counts, blood cultures, metabolic panels, D-dimer, lactic acid, and procalcitonin levels; monitor cardiac performance; monitor blood pressure; give oxygen to maintain pulse oxygen >94; monitor waveform capnography; and administer Tylenol, IV fluids, vasopressors, corticosteroids, and antibiotics as ordered. **Pronation position** prior to and after intubation has been helpful in improving pulse oximetry levels. If intubation is needed, use N95 mask, full PPE, and negative pressure room. **A high efficiency particulate air (HEPA) filter** attached to the bag valve mask (BVM) or endotracheal tube should be utilized if intubation or rescue breathing necessary.

Notes: ____

RADIATION

Radiation is a natural or manufactured form of energy that can be dangerous at high levels of exposure. Sometimes radiation exposure is combined with other disasters. For example, the 2011 and 2016 earthquake–tsunami combination in Japan caused a nuclear power plant to melt down.

- *Causes:* High-level exposures from sources such as a terrorist attack or nuclear power plant accident.
- *Signs and symptoms:* Burns; nausea, vomiting, and diarrhea; weakness; bleeding; confusion; sepsis; or symptom free.
- *Interventions:* Provide medical personnel with radiation detection devices; use reverse isolation/neutropenic precautions; anticipate orders to obtain a complete blood count, provide trauma/burn care, administer fluids intravenously, and give nausea medications and iodide tablets.

Notes: ____

Question: An A&E patient significantly exposed to radiation on the job will have which symptoms?

Answer: *Bloody diarrhea, nausea, and vomiting within 3 hours of radiation exposure.*

SMALLPOX

Smallpox is a viral infection (*Variola major*).

- *Causes:* Spread by prolonged face-to-face contact; direct contact; or an exchange of bodily fluids.
- *Signs and symptoms:* Two to 3 days of fever; fatigue; nausea and vomiting; and delirium. This is followed by an approximately 4- to 6-mm macular rash on the face and extremities that turn to papules, vesicles, pustules, and finally scars (see Figure 5.3).
- *Interventions:* Take **airborne and contact precautions**; place patient in negative-pressure room; contact the CDC for laboratory testing and wound care; and give smallpox vaccination as ordered.

Notes: ____

Essential Facts

Smallpox has been successfully eradicated as a result of multinational vaccinations. Because people are no longer vaccinated, there is concern that the *V. major* virus could be used as a bioterrorism weapon affecting our younger generations, born after 1980.

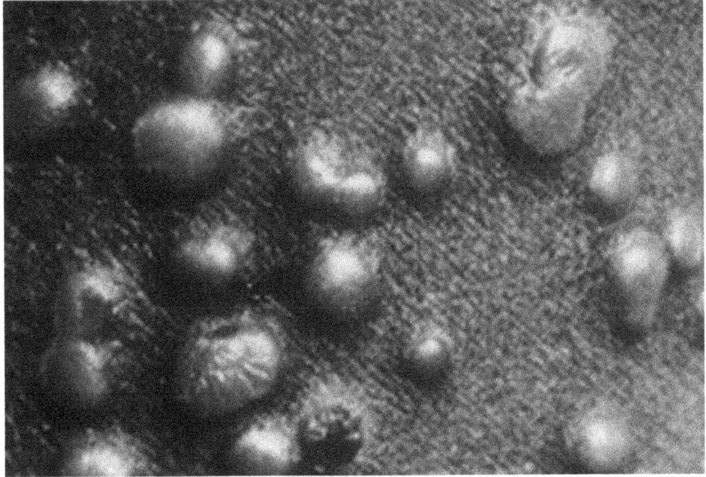

Figure 5.3 Smallpox rash.
Source: www.cdc.gov/smallpox/symptoms/index.html

TULAREMIA

Tularemia is a gram-negative bacterial infection (*Franciscella tularensis*).

- *Causes:* Spread by contact with infected animals, biting flies, or ticks.
- *Signs and symptoms:* Within 2 weeks, the patient may experience abdominal pain; fever; nausea, vomiting, and diarrhea; pneumonia; conjunctivitis; skin ulcer; and lymphadenitis.
- *Interventions:* Maintain standard precautions; gather blood, wound, or sputum cultures; and give antibiotics (ciprofloxacin, doxycycline, and gentamicin) as ordered.

Notes: ____

VIRAL HEMORRHAGIC FEVERS

Rare but deadly viral hemorrhagic fevers include infections, such as **Ebola**, Marburg, and yellow fever.

- *Causes:* Spread by inhalation, direct contact or consuming infected animal (bats, monkeys, and apes), or direct human contact or bodily fluid exchange.
- *Signs and symptoms:* Within 3 weeks, the patient experiences fever; headache; weakness; body aches; diarrhea; vomiting blood; bleeding gums; petechial rash; jaundice; bruising; hemorrhaging; hematuria; nose bleeds; disseminated intravascular coagulation; hepatitis; and renal failure.
- *Interventions:* Identify, Isolate, and Inform. **Document travel history in past 21 days**; establish airborne/contact precautions; place patient in negative-pressure room; inform the hospital infection preventionist and the CDC. **Scene safety always comes first**. Medical personnel minimally require surgical mask, face shield, fluid-resistant gown, and double gloves with extended cuffs. A full-body PPE and personal air-purifying respirators may be necessary for patients with advanced/severe symptoms according to policy. *Take your time* to **ensure proper donning and doffing techniques for highly infectious diseases using a buddy system and equipment checklist**. Visit the CDC website to view recommended web-based PPE training. The virus can live outside the body on dry surfaces for hours and in room-temperature body fluids for days. Anticipate orders to obtain a

complete blood count, liver function tests, prothrombin/partial thromboplastin time, and enzyme-linked immunosorbent assay (ELISA) testing; antiemetics; antipyretics; IV fluids; vasopressors; provide supportive treatment; and give antivirals, such as arenavirus, regeneron, or ribavirin. Only yellow fever and Zaire Ebola vaccines are currently available, but the infection may take over before the vaccine is effective.

Notes: ____

CHOLERA (*VIBRIO CHOLERAE*)

Cholera, an intestinal infection caused by the bacterium *V. cholerae*, is uncommon in the United States, but may occur in individuals who return home after travel to Africa, India, or South America. Its severe effects can be life-threatening, from rapid loss of body fluids and shock. It is estimated that 95,000 people die annually from cholera.

- *Causes:* Spreads through ingested fecal-contaminated water or food.
- *Signs and symptoms:* Severe watery diarrhea and vomiting; leg cramps; dehydration; and shock.
- *Interventions:* Maintain standard precautions; anticipate orders to perform a complete blood count and basic metabolic panel; provide fluid bolus intravenously; and possibly give antibiotics and zinc supplements.

Notes: ____

DISASTER AFTER CARE

Dependent on the size and severity of the disaster, staff may exhibit anxiety, depression, loss of concentration, inability to sleep, or other symptoms of posttraumatic stress. Critical incident stress debriefing is often helpful to allow staff to talk about their experience and offer tips for coping. Debriefing can be conducted by anyone; however, trained facilitators may have better results.

SUMMARY

Disasters are rarely predictable and are always chaotic. You will need to remain calm, stay informed, and **be flexible** as your entire day-to-day routines and procedures may change rapidly. The hospital may run out of certain supplies and resources; you may have to be good stewards of the supplies you have and use whatever is available. It is critical that you be prepared and know the various action plans for your facility. Become familiar with all available disaster equipment. Although this chapter should give you a good working knowledge of common forms of disasters and what to do, participating in disaster drills is an essential piece of the puzzle. Be sure to routinely refresh your disaster-nursing skills by **actively participating in regional drills and exercises.**

6

Endocrine Emergencies

The endocrine system is made up of several complex hormone-secreting glands. These include the pituitary, pineal gland, hypothalamus, parathyroid, thyroid, pancreas, adrenals, testes, and ovaries. When one thinks of the endocrine system, the word that might come to mind is "hormones." While the endocrine system is responsible for hormone production, it also affects metabolism, growth and development, emotions, tissue function, and homeostasis. Although there are many endocrine-related illnesses, this chapter includes only the most common and emergent. After reviewing this chapter, you will be able to differentiate the different types of endocrine emergencies and their causes, manifestations, and treatments.

During this part of your orientation, locate and become familiar with:

- Blood glucose monitoring devices
- Diabetic ketoacidosis (DKA) policy and procedure
- Hypoglycemia protocol and procedure
- Dietary supplies in your A&E
- Medications to know: insulin, insulin drips, antipyretics, beta-blockers, iodides and propylthiouracil (PTU), oral and intravenous (IV) potassium, sodium bicarbonate, IV calcium, IV dextrose, glucagon, sodium polystyrene sulfonate (Kayexalate), and albuterol

The pancreas is located in the mid-upper abdomen and is responsible for production and secretion of insulin and digestive enzymes such as amylase and lipase.

DIABETIC KETOACIDOSIS

DKA is a state of metabolic acidosis that is the result of elevated blood sugar (>250 mg/dL). When the blood sugar is this high, the body does not have sufficient insulin to break down sugar for energy. To compensate, the body breaks down fat, thereby releasing toxic ketone acids.

- *Causes:* Uncontrolled blood sugar in diabetes mellitus, pancreatitis, illness, infection, stress, pregnancy, and alcohol or drug abuse.
- *Signs and symptoms:* Dry, flushed skin; serum glucose level >250 mg/dL; nausea and vomiting; abdominal pain; increased thirst; tachycardia; hypotension; urinary frequency; weakness; fruity breath; Kussmaul breathing; ketones in urine; change in level of consciousness; and coma. Onset of symptoms is typically 2 to 3 days.
- *Interventions:*
  - *Fluid replacement:* Administer IV normal saline bolus. Use caution if patient has a history of congestive heart failure or renal failure. Once you replace fluids, be prepared for urinary frequency. Provide urinals or bedpans. Collect urinalysis looking for ketones and glucose and monitor intake and output.
  - *Correct acidosis:* Check arterial or venous blood gases per policy; obtain beta-hydroxybutyrate (BHB) levels; monitor pulse oximetry or waveform capnography; administer IV sodium bicarbonate if ordered.
  - *Balance electrolytes:* Monitor anion gap, metabolic panel every 2 to 4 hours, and cardiac rhythm; give nothing by mouth (NPO); medicate for nausea and vomiting. Anticipate IV potassium orders for hypokalemia. *Insulin administration drives potassium back into the cells, further reducing serum potassium levels.* Monitor potassium levels every 1 to 2 hours.
  - *Treat hyperglycemia:* Obtain and monitor **hourly blood glucose**, acetone level, and urinalysis; give insulin (first, 5–10 units of regular IV push, and then 0.1 units/kg/hr by IV

fusion on a pump). Once the patient's blood sugar is <200 to 250 mg/dL, typically a **subcutaneous (SQ) insulin dose is ordered to be given 2 hours prior to discontinuing the IV insulin drip.** This allows for a smooth transition from IV to SQ insulin. IV 5% dextrose 0.45% normal saline (D5½NS) at a rate of 150 to 200 mL/hr may be ordered as serum sodium returns to normal and glucose levels reach ≤250 mg/dL. Prepare for ICU admission.

Notes: ____

Question: A 29-year-old diabetic female arrives who has dried skin, is flushed, is hot, and has Kussmaul respirations. What is the underlying illness?
Answer: *DKA—check her blood sugar.*

Question: When is DKA considered resolved?
Answer: *When the serum pH is >7.3, serum bicarbonate level is ≥15 mEq/L, blood glucose is <200 mg/dL, and anion gap is ≤12; corrections should be gradual to avoid cerebral edema.*

Question: How often should you check blood sugars on a patient receiving an insulin IV drip?
Answer: *Every hour.*

HYPEROSMOLAR HYPERGLYCEMIC SYNDROME

This is a severe state of dehydration as a result of a very high blood sugar count (>600 mg/dL, but usually in the 1,000s). It is commonly associated with type 2 diabetes, recent surgery, medications, or illness.

- *Causes:* Uncontrolled diabetes, recent injury, illness, infection, stress, or medications cause a gradual rise in blood sugar over five or more days. The body tries to eliminate the excess sugar through frequent urination. Excess sugar and fluids are excreted repeatedly until the patient is left in a severely dehydrated state.
- *Signs and symptoms:* Imagine a shriveled, dried-up raisin, as this is your patient with hyperosmolar hyperglycemic syndrome (HHS)! Look for thirst; warm and dry skin; dry mucosa; urinary

frequency; weakness; change in level of consciousness; seizures; tachycardia; hypotension; fever; and absence of ketones in urine.

- *Interventions:*
  - *Fluid replacement:* These patients may need up to 9 to 12 L of IV fluids. Anticipate orders to start with normal saline IV bolus over 1 to 2 hours. Increased bolus rate may be ordered if hypotension is present. Frequently document vital signs. Use caution if patient has a history of congestive heart failure or renal failure. Once you replace fluids, be prepared for urinary frequency. Provide urinals or bedpans. Collect urinalysis and monitor intake and output.
  - *Balance electrolytes:* Monitor serum osmolality, metabolic panel, and cardiac rhythm; obtain EKG; keep NPO; medicate for nausea and vomiting. Anticipate IV potassium orders for hypokalemia. *Insulin administration drives potassium back into the cells, further reducing serum potassium levels.*
  - *Treat hyperglycemia:* Obtain and **monitor blood glucose hourly**, acetone level, and urinalysis; give insulin (5–10 units of regular IV push, and then 0.05 units/kg/hr by IV fusion on a pump until blood sugar is <300 mg/dL). The goal is to slowly reduce serum glucose by 50 to 70 mg/dL/hr; rapid reduction can cause cerebral edema. This happens over several days and will take several days to gradually reverse. Once the patient's blood sugar is <200 to 300 mg/dL, change from IV to SQ insulin per the provider's order. IV 5% dextrose 0.45% normal saline (D5½NS) at a rate of 150 to 200 mL/hr may be ordered as serum sodium returns to normal and glucose levels reach ≤250 mg/dL. Prepare for possible ICU admission.

Notes: ____

Essential Facts

Note the symptom and blood sugar differences between HHS and DKA.

- HHS means that blood sugar is very high (600–1,000s mg/dL). It is more common in type 2 diabetics or diet-controlled diabetics who don't often check their blood sugar. Patient is severely dehydrated, serum pH is normal, and there are *no* **ketones** in the urine.
- DKA blood sugar is moderately high (250–600 mg/dL). It is more common in type 1 diabetics or new onset. Fruity breath odor may be noted. The patient may be mildly dehydrated, arterial blood gas (ABGs) reveal acidosis, and **ketones are present** in the urine.

HYPOGLYCEMIA

Hypoglycemia is defined as a low blood sugar (<60–70 mg/dL) and most commonly affects type 1 diabetics.

- *Causes:* Taking too much insulin or diabetic medication; lack of food intake; pancreatic tumor; sepsis; stress; pregnancy; alcohol ingestion; adrenal insufficiency; liver disease; and certain medications such as beta-blockers, nonsteroidal anti-inflammatory drugs (NSAIDs), and thyroid hormones.
- *Signs and symptoms:* Anxiety; hunger; sweating; dry mouth; pallor; altered mental status; confusion; lethargy; headache; hypothermia; **loss of consciousness;** and death.
- *Interventions:* Obtain accurate history, complete neurologic assessment, and assess for cause of hypoglycemia. Anticipate orders to obtain blood glucose, monitor cardiac rhythm and vital signs, provide warm blankets and warming measures if hypothermic, obtain IV access, obtain complete blood count and metabolic panel, and recheck the blood glucose in 1 hour of treatment and as needed.
    - *If conscious:* Anticipate orders to give simple carbohydrates orally in the form of orange juice, soda, or glucose gel to quickly raise the blood sugar. Then give the patient a sandwich meal or regular diet tray to provide complex carbohydrates that will sustain the blood sugar.
    - *If unconscious:* Anticipate orders to give IV dextrose or intramuscular glucagon if unable to obtain IV access. Once patient regains consciousness, give simple carbohydrates followed by complex carbohydrates. *Vomiting may occur after glucagon administration; consider aspiration precautions.*

Notes: ____

PANCREATITIS

This is the result of an increase in pancreatic enzymes. Whether it is caused by overproduction or obstruction, the enzymes erode or eat away the pancreatic tissues. Pancreatitis can spread to the liver, diaphragm, lungs, and other nearby organs. It is basically the **pancreas in self-destruct or autodigestion mode.** This inflammation can spread rapidly leading to Systemic Inflammatory Response Syndrome **(SIRS).**

- *Causes:* Use the mnemonic **GET SMASHED:** Gallstones, Ethanol, Trauma, Steroids, Mumps, Autoimmune disorders, Scorpion stings, Hyperlipidemia/hypercalcemia, Endoscopic retrograde cholangio-pancreatography (ERCP), and **Dr**ug toxicity. Contributing factors include smoking, stress, and crash dieting or binge eating.
- *Signs and symptoms:* Midepigastric abdominal pain radiating to the back; hypocalcemia; diminished bowel sounds; nausea and vomiting; abdominal distention; low-grade fever; jaundice if gallstones; weight loss; tachycardia; hypotension; **frothy, fatty, and foul-smelling stools**; dark urine; Grey Turner's sign (see Figure 6.1); Cullen's sign (see Figure 6.2); and altered blood sugar.
- *Interventions:* Anticipate orders to administer fluids intravenously; monitor **serum amylase, serum lipase,** liver enzymes, and blood glucose level; use nasogastric tube for decompression; administer nothing NPO; give medications (antacids, anticholinergics, histamine receptor agonists, insulin, nitroglycerin, antispasmodics, and analgesics/narcotics); prevent and treat infections; prepare for ultrasound or CT; prepare for possible surgery; and instruct patient on diet (low-fat diet, no caffeine, and no alcohol).

Notes: ____

Question: What is the normal serum amylase level in adults younger than 60 years?
Answer: *25 to 125 U/L.*

The patient who is actively vomiting cannot drink water before seeing the A&E provider *in case the patient ends up going to surgery.*

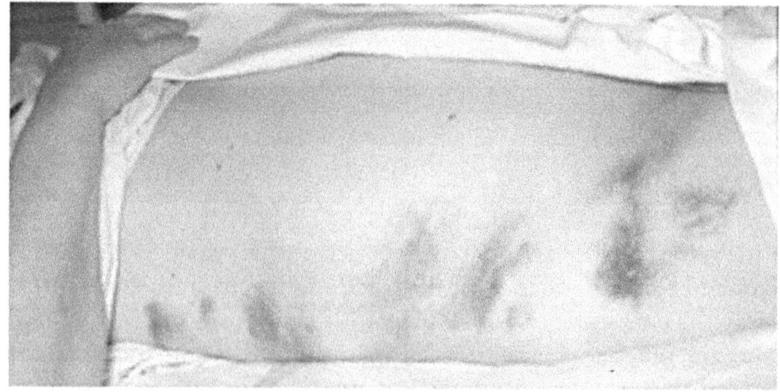

Figure 6.1 Grey Turner's sign.
Source: Herbert L. Fred and Hendrik A. van Dijk.

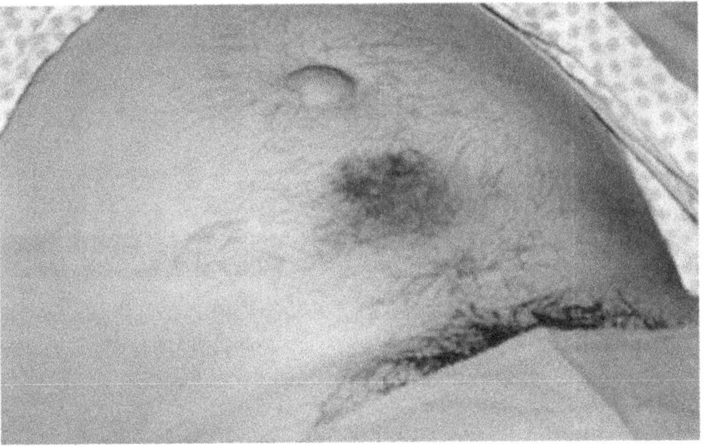

Figure 6.2 Cullen's sign.
Source: Herbert L. Fred and Hendrik A. van Dijk.

THYROID-RELATED EMERGENCIES

The thyroid is located in the anterior aspect of the neck and affects calcium metabolism. Thyroid emergencies are rare but can be life threatening.

THYROID STORM

Thyroid storm is a life-threatening emergency that results from poorly managed hyperthyroidism.

- *Causes:* Uncontrolled hyperthyroidism. Risk factors include history of Graves' disease, medication noncompliance, thyroid tumors, certain medications (amiodarone, lithium) trauma, infection, childbirth, recent surgery, illness, or stress.
- *Signs and symptoms:* Vary but may include high fever; tachycardia; hypertension; vomiting; diarrhea; jaundice; thinning hair; weight loss; sweating; restlessness; exophthalmos; goiter; and tremors.
- *Interventions:* Obtain accurate history and list of medications; promptly manage any airway, breathing, and circulation concerns first; and provide supportive care. Anticipate orders to administer antipyretics, beta-blockers (propranolol), iodides, and

PTU; obtain IV access; obtain serum thyroid function, metabolic panel, complete blood count, and toxicology screen; apply cooling blankets for targeted temperature management; give supplemental oxygen; and obtain CT of head.

Notes: ____

Essential Facts

A patient in thyroid storm may appear almost toxic with extremely high fevers reaching as high as 103 °F to 105 °F. Treatment should be aggressive, as this is a life-threatening emergency!

MYXEDEMA COMA

Myxedema coma is a rare but emergent complication of uncontrolled or undiagnosed hypothyroidism. It is more common in women than in men and occurs more often in the winter months.

- *Causes:* Hashimoto's disease; iodine deficiency; pituitary dysfunction; tumor; medications such as lithium, beta-blockers, amiodarone, narcotics, interferon, anticonvulsants, and general anesthesia; stress; burns; infection; surgery; trauma; and hypothermia.
- *Signs and symptoms:* Fatigue; shortness of breath; weight gain; tongue swelling; generalized edema; constipation; pale cool skin; multiple organ dysfunction; hypothermia; bradycardia; bradypnea; confusion; depression; decreased urinary output; possible hypoglycemia; altered mental status or psychosis; coma; respiratory failure; and death.
- *Interventions:* Support airway, breathing, and circulation. Anticipate orders to obtain IV access; complete blood count, thyroid levels, metabolic panel, and serum creatinine levels; have EKG; administer IV or oral levothyroxine (Synthroid); slowly and passively rewarm patient; monitor intake and output; and administer analgesics and glucocorticoids.

Notes: ____

Essential Facts

Be sure to closely monitor the cardiac rhythm of a myxedema coma patient. EKG findings associated with myxedema coma include bundle branch blocks, complete heart blocks, ST segment and T-wave changes, and bradycardia with prolonged QT intervals.

Question: Prolonged QT intervals can be a precursor for which type of arrhythmias?

Answer: *Ventricular tachycardia and torsades de pointes.*

SUMMARY

Those little hormones can affect so much more than just your mood. The endocrine system can **affect multiple body systems**. If you have ever been pregnant, you may have experienced firsthand how much hormones can affect the rest of the body. Document a full primary assessment, all interventions, and any hourly blood glucose results. Do not infuse insulin if serum potassium is <3.3. Early recognition, thorough assessment, and rapid treatment are crucial to the survival of an endocrine-related emergency.

7

Environmental Emergencies

Let us face it: Potential environmental hazards are all around us. The love of outdoor sports and activities contributes to the risks of environmental emergencies. Caring for the environmentally ill or injured patient is a common occurrence in the A&E. This chapter guides you through the many common types of environmental challenges you may face. Because no two environments are quite the same, be sure to become familiar with the most common environmental emergencies in your area.

During this part of your orientation, locate and become familiar with:

- Local and state animal bite-reporting regulations
- Wound cleansing or irrigation materials
- Tetanus vaccination policy and procedures
- Rabies vaccination policy and procedures
- Local and state assault-reporting procedures
- Venomous creatures indigenous to your area
- Poisonous plants indigenous to your area
- Hemostatic dressing material
- Operating room (OR) admission process
- Warming equipment
- Cooling equipment

ANIMAL BITES

The most common animal bites seen in the A&E are dog or cat bites. Occasionally, you may encounter a patient with a raccoon, rodent, or rabbit bite. Dog bites can exert a pressure of 200 to 450 lb per square inch (PSI) resulting in more tissue damage, whereas cat bites pose a higher risk for infection.

- *Causes:* Break in the skin or tissue damage related to bite injury from an animal.
- *Signs and symptoms:* May range from lacerations, puncture wounds, to crush or soft-tissue injuries.
- *Interventions:* **Report all animal bites to your local animal control** health authority. Assess wounds, noting any deformities or signs of infection. Anticipate orders to irrigate the wound with copious amounts of saline; administer antibiotics for high-risk injuries; administer rabies vaccine (only if the patient is unable to locate and quarantine the animal for 10 days); and administer tetanus vaccine if not vaccinated within past 5 years.

Notes: ____

Question: Which animal bite has the greatest risk for infection: dog, cat, or rat?
Answer: *Cat, because cats come in more contact with bacteria-infected rodents and create small puncture wounds.*

Question: A 36-year-old female comes in complaining of being bitten by a mouse. Should you give a rabies vaccine?
Answer: *No, small rodents do not carry rabies. However, skunks, foxes, raccoons, coyotes, dogs, cats, and bats may carry rabies.*

Question: If actually contracted, is rabies fatal without proper vaccination?
Answer: *Yes.*

BROWN RECLUSE SPIDER BITES

Brown recluse spiders are light brown with a darker brown, violin-shaped mark on their backs (see Figure 7.1). Spider bites are actually pretty rare. Most spiders bite only when threatened. Nevertheless, many A&E patients arrive almost daily, mistaking a common staph infection for a spider bite. Brown recluse spiders typically are found in the Midwestern and Southeastern parts of the United States.

- *Causes:* Bite from a brown recluse spider.
- *Signs and symptoms:* The initial bite is usually **painless**. Brown recluse venom is cytotoxic and hemolytic. Basically, a bite from this spider may result in tissue necrosis. Most commonly, your patient will experience only some erythema and pain at the site. Rarely, the erythema then develops a red or bluish blood-filled blister. When this blister ruptures, it leaves a necrotic ulcer.
- *Interventions:* Anticipate orders to cleanse and dress the affected area and administer prophylactic antibiotics, analgesics, steroids, dapsone, and tetanus vaccine. Most brown recluse bites heal without any medical attention. However, a small percentage of patients may develop a secondary infection, systemic inflammatory response, coagulopathies, renal failure, and death in small children.

Notes: ____

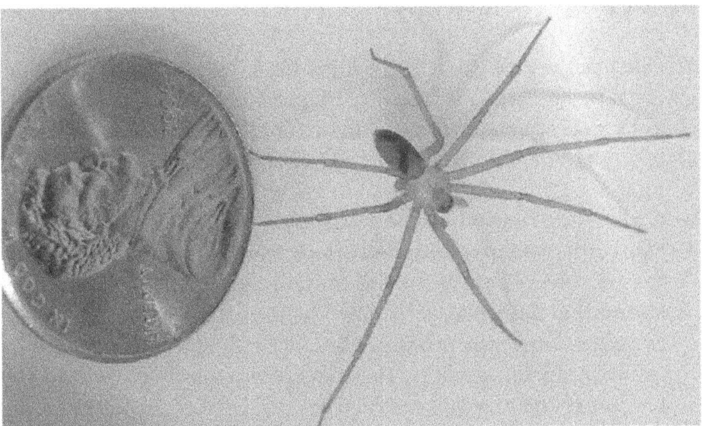

Figure 7.1 Brown recluse spider.
Source: Emmanuel Boutet.

The bite of a brown recluse spider may cause skin ulcers (see Figure 7.2). An easy way to remember this is to spell "ulcer" backward!

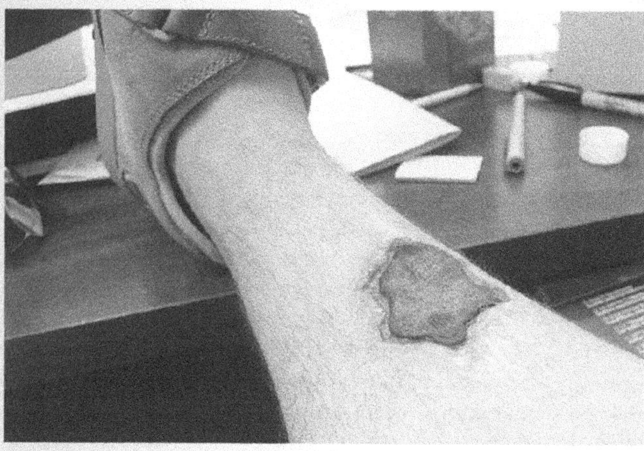

Figure 7.2 Skin ulcer.
Source: Jeffery Rowland.

BLACK WIDOW SPIDER BITES

Female black widow spiders are shiny black with a bright red hourglass mark on their abdomen (see Figure 7.3). Although the black widow's potent venom is neurotoxic, fatalities are rare. Children, older adults, and cardiac patients are more at risk.

- *Causes:* Bite from a black widow spider.
- *Signs and symptoms:* **Muscle cramps**; muscle contractions or spasms; **severe pain** at the site, musculoskeletal pain; **severe abdominal pain** similar to appendicitis; nausea; vomiting; hypertension; fever; weakness; headache; fatigue; anxiety; restlessness; and seizures. These symptoms may begin within a few hours and may last several days.
- *Interventions:* Treatment is usually supportive. Stabilize any airway, breathing, or circulation concerns first. Consult poison

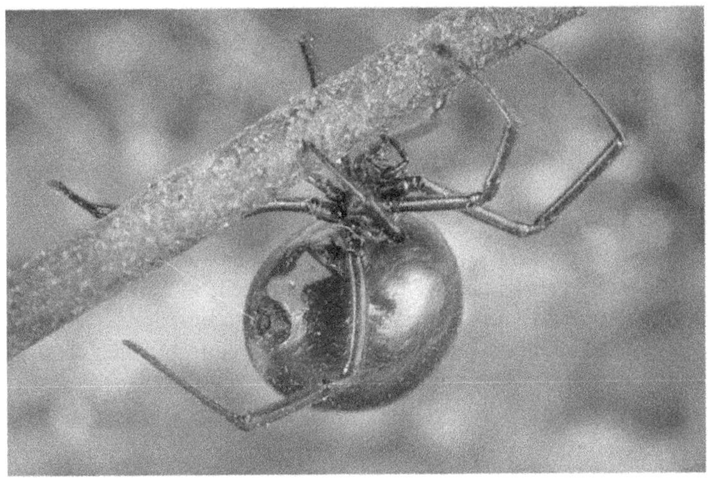

Figure 7.3 Black widow spider.
Source: Paula Smith/Centers for Disease Control and Prevention Public Health Image Library.

control and apply ice to the bite area to slow action of the venom. Anticipate orders to administer calcium gluconate, narcotics, muscle relaxants, antivenom skin test, and antivenom with antihistamines, if negative skin test.

Notes: ____

CROCODILE AND ALLIGATOR BITES

Alligator and crocodiles are found in Africa, Asia, South America, Australia, and the southern United States.

- *Causes:* Bites from alligators or crocodiles typically produce crushing, de-gloving injuries with multiple puncture wounds. In addition, a wide variety of bacteria can be found in the mouth of an alligator or crocodile. Therefore, these bites carry a high risk for infection.
- *Signs and symptoms:* Deep, severe soft-tissue crush and de-gloving injury with multiple puncture wounds. Patient may also arrive with limb amputation and in a state of hemorrhagic or hypovolemic shock.

- *Interventions:* Assess and treat any uncontrolled external hemorrhage with direct pressure, hemolytic and/or compression dressings, and, if severe, tourniquets. Stabilize airway, breathing, and circulation issues. Anticipate orders to obtain two large-bore intravenous (IV) accesses; complete blood count (CBC) with differential, blood cultures, wound cultures, and type and crossmatch. Other orders may include administration of multiple broad-spectrum IV antibiotics, intramuscular tetanus prophylaxis, IV crystalloid fluids, x-rays, splinting of deformed or fractured extremities, wound care/debridement, O-negative blood transfusion, and preparation for OR admission. Document repeated circulatory assessment findings before and after each intervention to determine effectiveness.

Notes: ____

HUMAN BITES

The human mouth carries more germs than that of most other animals. Therefore, a human bite is usually at a higher risk for infection than most animal bites.

- *Causes:* Bite from a human. You may see this if your patient was assaulted.
- *Signs and symptoms:* Bite marks to the skin resulting in puncture wounds, lacerations, soft-tissue damage, crush injury, and, rarely, amputation.
- *Interventions:* Anticipate orders to irrigate, cleanse, and dress wound and administer prophylactic antibiotics such as Augmentin (amoxicillin clavulanate). Report assaults to your local police department according to your state law.

Notes: ____

LIZARD BITES

- *Causes:* Bite from a lizard. Most lizard bites are nontoxic. However, Gila monsters (see Figure 7.4) and Mexican bearded lizards are venomous. These two lizards are commonly found in the southwestern United States and northwestern Mexico.
- *Signs and symptoms:* The bite may cause tissue trauma and crush injuries. The venom may produce pain, swelling, edema, nausea, vomiting, weakness, hemorrhage, tachycardia, hypotension, respiratory failure, syncope, shock, and possibly anaphylaxis.

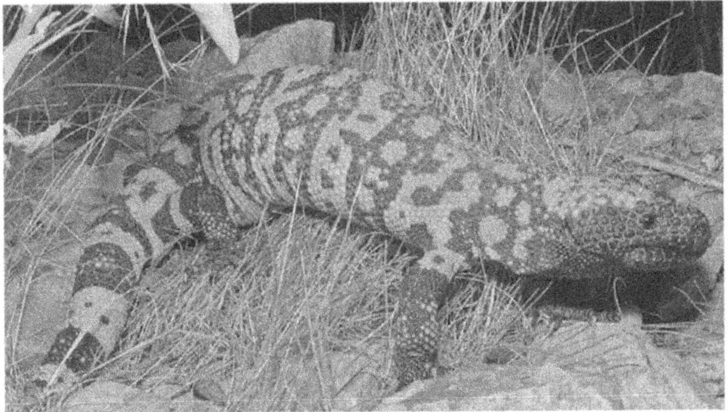

Figure 7.4 Gila monster.
Source: U.S. Fish & Wildlife Service, Arizona Ecological Services.

- *Interventions:* Lizard antivenom currently does not exist. Stabilize any airway, breathing, or circulation problems first. Anticipate orders for wound care, administration of analgesics and tetanus prophylaxis, and supportive care.

Notes: ____

SHARK BITES

- *Causes:* Bite from a shark. Most shark attack victims are taken by surprise and do not actually see what bit them. They often describe the attack as a sudden "tug" on an extremity. If you are working in an A&E near the coastline, you need to be prepared to manage this injury.
- *Signs and symptoms:* Abrasions if the shark bumps the victim first; crescent-shaped bites; puncture wounds; shark teeth fragments; parallel scrapes or lacerations; bone fractures; tissue loss; amputations; hypothermia; and hypotension related to severe blood loss. (See also signs and symptoms of hypovolemic shock in Chapter 21, Shock Emergencies.)
- *Interventions:* Assess and control any external hemorrhaging first with direct pressure, hemostatic and/or pressure dressings, or a tourniquet, if severe. Stabilize airway, breathing, and circulation. Provide warmth and apply oxygen. Anticipate orders to start two large-bore IV accesses, obtain blood type and crossmatch for possible blood transfusion, transfuse O-negative blood, and

prepare for possible OR admission. Document repeated circulatory assessment findings before and after each intervention to determine effectiveness.

Notes: ____

SNAKEBITES

Contrary to what is shown in many movies, snakes are not usually aggressive creatures. They usually bite only if provoked or threatened. Snakes can be either venomous or nonvenomous. In the United States, there are only two types of venomous snakes: the pit vipers (rattlesnakes, copperheads, and cottonmouths) and the elapidaes (coral snakes). Coral snake venom is neurotoxic, whereas pit viper venom is hemotoxic.

Essential Facts

To quickly tell the difference between venomous and nonvenomous snakes, look at the shapes of their heads (see Figure 7.5). The rattlesnake on the left has a more triangular-shaped head than the nonvenomous garter snake on the right, which has a narrow round-shaped head.

a) b)

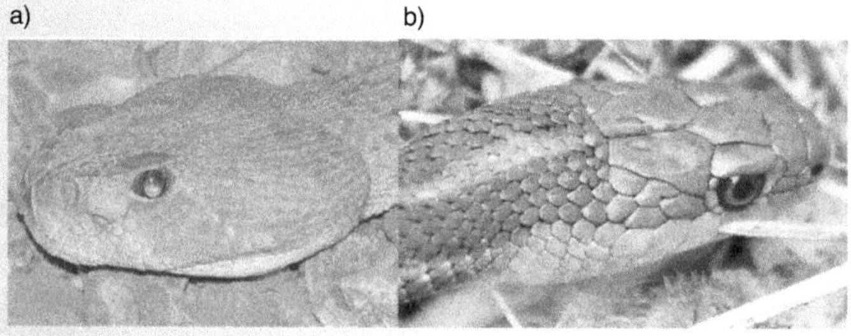

Figure 7.5 (a) Rattlesnake and (b) garter snake.
Source: Photo on right by Linda Tanner.

Coral snakes are a little tricky (see Figure 7.6). You cannot really tell if they are venomous by the shape of the head. However, there is a rhyme some use to remember; it is based on the snake's bright red and yellow bands of color. "Red touching yellow kills a fellow." Or if "red touches black, venom lack."

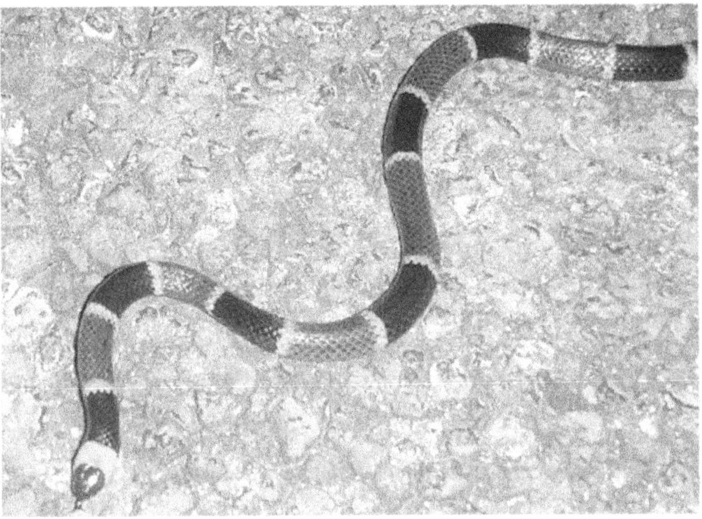

Figure 7.6 Coral snake.
Source: National Park Service.

The first snakebite patient I cared for was a 6-year-old girl who was bitten by a baby copperhead. I saw firsthand how a snake could "play dead." When the adult accompanying the child poured the "dead" snake out of a coffee cup onto the counter, it began to wiggle all over the place. We could tell it was a baby copperhead right away by its bright green tail. The greatest concern with baby snakes is that they have not yet learned how to control the release of their venom. They are more likely to deliver all their venom in one bite, whereas the adult can control how much, if any, venom should be released. In this case, the child received a full dose of venom to her ankle. Due to her progressive systemic symptoms, she had to receive antivenom.

- *Causes:* Bite from a venomous snake.
- *Signs and symptoms:* Life-threatening reactions may include hypovolemic shock, respiratory failure, renal failure, and severe hemorrhage. Depending on the type of snake, your patient may experience the following:
  - *Local:* Bleeding; one or two puncture marks; redness; swelling; edema; tissue damage; possible tissue necrosis; and pain at the site.
  - *Systemic:* Nausea; vomiting; diarrhea; increased thirst; dizziness; diaphoresis; fever; syncope; paralysis; excessive salivation; speech difficulties; metallic or rubber taste; muscle

twitching, paresthesia; gastric or rectal bleeding; epistaxis; hemoptysis; tachycardia; constricted pupils; oral swelling; abdominal pain; seizure; ecchymosis; petechiae; and weak pulse.

- *Interventions:* Stabilize airway, breathing, and circulation concerns first. Obtain an accurate history, including description of the snake, any treatment prior to arrival, time of bite, location, and number of bites. If the patient was bitten on their leg or arm, then immobilize affected limb at or **below heart level** and minimize exertion to reduce blood flow. Use a ballpoint pen or medical marker to mark a border of advancing edema every 15 minutes. Remove any jewelry or clothing from the bitten area. Anticipate orders to monitor cardiac rhythm, check blood pressure frequently, obtain large-bore IV access, administer IV crystalloid fluid bolus, administer analgesics for pain, administer tetanus prophylaxis, x-ray the affected area to reveal imbedded teeth, and obtain labs from unaffected arm (CBC, electrolytes, blood urea nitrogen, creatinine, creatine phosphokinase levels, and type and crossmatch). Due to the cost and risk of anaphylactic reaction, antivenom is not usually given prophylactically. The provider may order an antivenom skin test first to see if the patient will have a reaction. If your patient develops worsening symptoms, coagulopathies, or major systemic reactions, such as hypotension or altered mental status, you may anticipate orders to administer antivenom such as CroFab. Keep anaphylactic medications or kits at the bedside when administering antivenom in case an anaphylactic reaction occurs.

Essential Facts

Snakebite Management Myths—Corrected

Do *not* place a tourniquet above the site. When a tourniquet is taken off, it may release a venom bolus into the circulation, leading to systemic reaction.

Do *not* cut an "X" over the bite area and suck the venom out. It has been proven ineffective and may result in secondary infection.

Do *not* drink alcohol. Although drinking alcohol may lessen the patient's pain, it also dilates blood vessels, which may circulate the venom throughout the body faster.

Do *not* ice the limb. Although it may slow the blood flow to the area, icing is commonly associated with loss of a limb after a snakebite.

Believe it or not, most of your snakebite victims will try to kill the snake and bring it to show you which type of snake bit them. Educate your patients that a description of the snake will be safer for everyone.

Notes: ____

COLD-RELATED INJURIES

FROSTBITE

- *Causes:* Exposure to extreme cold. Increased risk factors include diabetes, heart disease, and alcohol consumption.
- *Signs and symptoms:* Vary depending on temperature and length of exposure. Extent of tissue damage may not be evident until several days after exposure. Typically, the ears, nose, fingers, cheeks, and toes are affected first.
  - *First degree or "frostnip":* Involves superficial skin surfaces, itching, pain, tingling, pallor, or red patches. There is no permanent tissue damage.
  - *Second degree:* Involves the skin and subcutaneous tissues, numbness, tingling, burning sensation, and stiff frozen skin. Upon thawing, frozen tissue may develop blisters, become mottled in color, and develop a hot stinging sensation.
  - *Third degree:* Involves muscles, tendons, ligaments, and bones. Tissue may be white or pale yellow and waxy in appearance; tissues are cold and hard with lack of sensation to affected areas. As tissue thaws, blisters, edema of the extremity, and black-gray mottling may occur before gangrenous necrosis develops.
- *Interventions:* Rewarm the patient, monitor core temperature, and immerse affected areas in warm (104 °F–110 °F) water. Anticipate orders to administer pain medication, warm IV fluids; administer tetanus vaccine if needed; apply a warming blanket or just warm blankets; avoid friction or pressure to affected areas; dress thawed tissues with soft bulky dressings for protection; and elevate the affected area to reduce swelling. Teach patient that damage initially looks worse before it looks better and the healing process may take several months, depending on the damage.

Notes: ____

Thawing of frozen tissue is very painful. Avoid rubbing or using friction to warm frostbitten tissue, as this will increase tissue damage.

HYPOTHERMIA

Hypothermia is defined as a core temperature <95 °F.

- *Causes:* Prolonged exposure to cold environment, submersion in cold water, and certain medical conditions such as hypoglycemia.
- *Signs and symptoms:* Shivering; weakness; slurred speech; confusion; weak pulses; bradycardia; dysrhythmias such as atrial or ventricular fibrillation; and bradypnea. Shivering stops at 86 °F/30 °C and below. An extra wave called the J or Osborn wave may be present right next to the S point on the EKG.
- *Interventions:* Anticipate orders to remove any wet clothing and dry the patient, cover the patient with warm dry blankets, monitor glucose levels, monitor core temperatures, monitor pulse oximetry and cardiac rhythm, increase room temperature, apply warming blanket or use warming equipment available, infuse warmed IV normal saline, and apply warmed, humidified oxygen. If severe hypothermia, anticipate orders to use more active measures, such as warm peritoneal lavage, esophageal rewarming tubes, warm bladder irrigations, warm gastrointestinal irrigation, hemodialysis, continuous arteriovenous rewarming, and extracorporeal rewarming cardiopulmonary bypass.

Notes: ____

Question: What is the appropriate method for warming a shivering patient with a core temperature of 95 °F (mild hypothermia)?

Answer: *Passive warming measures, such as warm environment, removal of wet clothes, and warm blankets.*

While you are trying to rewarm the hypothermic patient, something called "rewarming shock" may occur. As the patient begins to warm, peripheral vasodilation may occur, causing hypotension. As the cold blood from the extremities returns to the heart, it may further drop the core temperature and irritate the ventricles. This may lead to atrial or ventricular fibrillation. Warm the core areas first to avoid rewarming shock.

Hypothermia may also cause oxygen to dissociate from hemoglobin, further reducing oxyhemoglobin concentrations.

NEAR DROWNING OR SUBMERSION EVENT

Near drowning is defined as surviving suffocation while submerged in a liquid. The term "drowning" results in death within 24 hours of a submersion event.

- *Causes:* Can be intentional or accidental. Drowning can also be secondary to a head/neck injury or cardiac event while in cold water. It is commonly seen in males and young children and toddlers.
- *Signs and symptoms:* May vary based on type of water or liquid, water temperature, length of submersion, concurrent injuries, and initiation of basic life support. Commonly you may see difficulty in breathing, tachypnea, or apnea, cold pale-blue or gray color skin, **hypoxia**, **acidosis,** bradycardia, hypotension, dilated pupils or "fish eyes," vomiting, and **hypothermia.**
- *Interventions:* Treat any airway, breathing, or circulation concerns first, maintaining C-spine immobilization, as C-spine injuries are common with diving accidents. Anticipate orders to apply oxygen via nonrebreather or bag valve mask; prepare for intubation if necessary; monitor core temperature; monitor cardiac rhythm; perform EKG; establish IV access; remove wet clothing and warm the patient; and obtain labs such as CBC, metabolic panel, and arterial blood gas.

Notes: ____

HEAT EXHAUSTION

- *Causes:* Prolonged exposure to warm temperatures and/or fluid loss without proper fluid and electrolyte replacement. If untreated, it may progress to heat stroke.
- *Signs and symptoms:* Extreme thirst; headache; dizziness; weakness; muscle cramps; nausea; vomiting; hypotension; tachycardia; fever; and syncope.
- *Interventions:* Place the patient on a stretcher and provide a cool, quiet area for the patient to rest. Anticipate orders to place the patient on a cardiac monitor, administer IV fluid bolus, monitor blood pressure and temperature, and continue with possible application of cooling blanket. Discharge teaching should include measures to avoid or prevent future heat exhaustion.

Notes: ____

HEAT STROKE

Heat stroke is a failure of the body to effectively dissipate heat and cool down. It is characterized by core temperatures over 105 °F and can be fatal despite aggressive treatment.

- *Causes:* Prolonged exposure to hot temperatures, usually in combination with dehydration or physical exertion. Heat stroke can occur if children are locked in vehicles on hot days. Infants and older adults are at increased risk. Risk factors include ingesting certain prescription or recreational drugs, preexisting medical conditions, high environmental temperatures, and high humidity.
- *Signs and symptoms:* Headache, dizziness, anxiety, and altered mental status; delirium; loss of muscle coordination; dilated/fixed pupils; seizures; hot, flushed, reddened, and dry skin; tachypnea; and coma.
- *Interventions:* Establish stable airway, breathing, and circulation first. Anticipate orders to apply oxygen, place patient on cardiac monitor, establish IV access, administer normal saline IV fluid bolus, cool the patient until core body temperature reaches 102 °F, monitor core temperature frequently, administer corticosteroids if cerebral edema occurs, monitor intake and output, and

prepare for possible ICU admission. Cooling by evaporation with moistened skin may be more effective than with dry skin and application of cooling blanket. Applying padded ice packs to vascular areas (groin, axilla, and neck) also helps to quickly reduce core temperatures. Your goal is to avoid shivering, as it will increase your patient's oxygen consumption. If shivering occurs, anticipate orders to give 10 to 15 mg of chlorpromazine (Thorazine) intravenously.

Notes: ____

HIGH-ALTITUDE ILLNESS OR ACUTE MOUNTAIN SICKNESS

As I researched material for this subject, my husband was preparing to hike Mount Whitney, the highest mountain in the continental United States. Although he and his friend did acclimate over a couple of days as they ascended, my husband still experienced signs of hypoxic stress. After the trip, he confessed his pulse oxygen levels were reading in the upper 80s during the hike. Thankfully, neither he nor his friend developed much pulmonary or cerebral edema on this particular trip. However, my husband has witnessed other hikers who did experience symptoms of high-altitude cerebral edema (HACE) and high-altitude pulmonary edema (HAPE).

High-altitude illness (HAI) or acute mountain sickness (AMS) is a hypoxia-related injury to high elevations (typically above 3,000 m or 9,800 ft). This can occur with mountain sports, air travel, or flight rescue work.

- *Causes:* Rapid ascent up high elevations without allowing the body to acclimate by spending days at an intermediate altitude. History of previous HAI, obesity, drug use, alcohol use, or other chronic lung or heart illness may predispose a person to HAI.
- *Signs and symptoms:* Headaches, dizziness, nausea, vomiting, **confusion**, pulse oxygen levels below 94%, pale skin, weakness, peripheral and facial edema, and **crackles/rales** may be auscultated over the chest.
- *Interventions:* The patient will need to descend to a lower elevation by at least 500 m or 1,640 ft. Assess and stabilize any airway, breathing, or circulation issues first. Once in the A&E, monitor pulse oxygen and capnography levels, document neurologic assessments, document respiratory findings; anticipate orders for chest x-ray or head CT; **provide supplemental**

oxygen to keep pulse oxygen above 94%, and keep patient warm. Anticipated orders to administer medications such as dexamethasone, ibuprofen, and acetazolamide. Hyperbaric treatment may be considered if available. Prepare for possible admission.

DECOMPRESSION SICKNESS

Decompression sickness can occur when diving. The deeper one dives the more water weight is exerted on the body. All this pressure compresses the gases inside the body especially nitrogen. As one surfaces, the weight of water on the body decreases and compressed gases in the body expand.

- *Causes:* Surfacing to quickly when diving. If nitrogen gases expand and enlarge too quickly, they can't cross the alveolar membrane to be exhaled thus becoming trapped inside the body. Trapped inside the nitrogen gas bubbles keep expanding and enlarging causing vascular occlusion and ischemia.
- *Signs and symptoms:* Cough, difficulty in breathing, headache, joint pain, jaw pain, facial pains, lethargy, paralysis, itchy paresthesia, blind spots, visual disturbances, altered mental status, loss of speech, inability to hear, and unconsciousness.
- *Interventions:* Anticipate orders to administer 100% oxygen via nonrebreather, IV fluids, nonnarcotic pain medications, and hyperbaric chamber treatment, if available.

Notes: ____

LIGHTNING INJURIES

Lightning strike injuries are a serious and potentially fatal injury. There are approximately 1,500 injuries that are reported each year with 25% of those being fatal.

- *Causes:* Contact with lighting either directly or indirectly.
- *Signs and symptoms:* Altered level of consciousness, apnea, dysrhythmias (inverted T wave, ST elevation, and prolonged QT interval), hypotension, cool skin, fixed dilated pupils, temporary paralysis, myoglobinuria, burns with entrance and exit wounds, and hearing loss. Lightning injuries have a high rate variability of complications due to the specific circumstances of the strike and the varying resistance of body tissues. Overall, the cardiovascular and nervous systems are most effected.

- *Interventions:* Anticipate orders to obtain cardiac monitoring, 12-lead EKG, CBC, electrolytes with blood urea nitrogen (BUN), creatinine, troponin, creatinine phosphokinase, and urinalysis; monitor for rhabdomyolysis, seizure precautions, chest x-ray, cervical spine x-ray, and head CT; and clean and dress burn wounds.

Notes: ____

Question: After airway breathing and circulation have been stabilized, what intervention would be of high priority for a lightning strike victim?

Answer: *Cardiac monitoring and 12-lead EKG. Due to the effects, a lightning strike can have on the cardiac system.*

STINGS

HYMENOPTERAN STINGS

Hymenopteran stings come from bees, fire ants, hornets, and wasps.

- *Causes:* Sting from hymenopteran venomous insects such as bees, fire ants, hornets, and wasps.
- *Signs and symptoms:* May vary from local reactions to severe systemic reactions depending on the location, number of stings, and patient sensitivity.
  - *Local:* Swelling, itching, redness, stinging, and burning.
  - *Systemic:* Edema, hives, bronchospasms, wheezing, and facial or oral swelling.
- *Interventions:* Treat any airway, breathing, or circulation problems first. Gently scrape stinger away with dull object (credit card), taking care not to squeeze the stinger, as it still contains some venom. Apply ice to site. Anticipate orders to administer antihistamines such as diphenhydramine (Benadryl) or famotidine (Pepcid), steroids such as methylprednisolone (Solumedrol), and, if severe, epinephrine 1:1,000 subcutaneously or intramuscularly. Many patients who develop allergic reactions to bee stings receive a prescription for an EpiPen. Discharge teaching on proper use of the EpiPen is vital to reduce future risks of mortality from anaphylaxis.

Notes: ____

> **Question:** When a patient arrives at the A&E for a bee sting, which symptoms would alert the nurse that the patient needs emergent management?
>
> **Answer:** *Angioedema, wheezing, or bronchospasms.*

JELLYFISH STINGS

- *Causes:* Sting from jellyfish. Be careful, because jellyfish that have washed ashore can still release venom.
- *Signs and symptoms:* Can be local or systemic and may vary based on size and type of jellyfish, duration of exposure, area of skin affected, age and health of the patient, and patient sensitivity.
  - *Local:* Instant stinging or burning; itching; tentacle print or patterned marks to the skin; numbness or tingling; and throbbing-type pain that may radiate up extremity. Jellyfish stings to the eye will require immediate eye irrigation and ophthalmology consult or follow-up.
  - *Systemic:* Headache; dizziness; fever; nausea; vomiting; muscle weakness; muscle spasm; joint pain; difficulty in breathing; arrhythmia; syncope; anaphylaxis; and cardiopulmonary arrest.
- *Interventions:* Treat any airway, breathing, or circulation problems first. Local reactions may be treated with rubbing alcohol, topical antihistamines, or corticosteroids. Anticipate orders to administer analgesics or topical anesthetics for pain, antihistamines, steroids, epinephrine, or, if box jellyfish, antivenom may be ordered.

Home remedies include rinsing the area with vinegar for at least 30 seconds to deactivate the venom. A paste made of seawater and baking soda has been known to deactivate venom of sea nettles and Portuguese man of war jellyfish. It is best to remove any tentacles with sea water, as freshwater may activate venom.

Notes: ____

SCORPION STINGS

Scorpions are found primarily in the southwestern region of the United States. There are many different types, but only one whose neurotoxic venom is considered lethal. This deadly scorpion is none

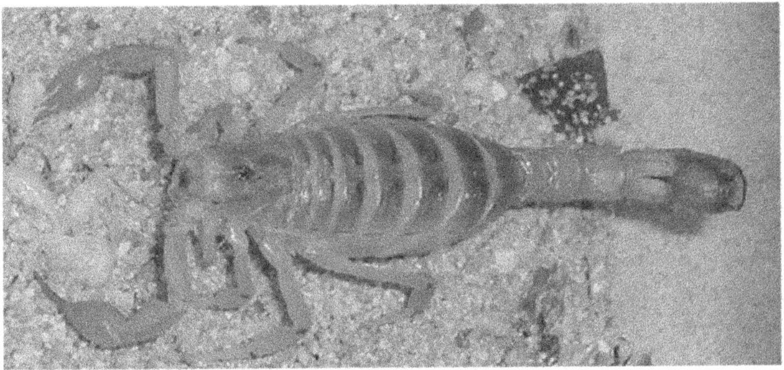

Figure 7.7 Scorpion.
Source: HDDuane.

other than the *Centruroides sculpturatus*, more commonly known as the "bark scorpion," as it dwells on tree bark (see Figure 7.7).

- *Causes:* Sting from the tail of a venomous scorpion.
- *Signs and symptoms:* Commonly local and rarely systemic.
  - *Local:* Instant pain; edema; swelling; redness; and numbness or tingling. These symptoms usually resolve without treatment in a few hours.
  - *Systemic:* Agitation; anxiety; impaired speech; visual disturbances; incontinence; tachypnea; wheezing; stridor; excessive salivation; jaw muscle spasms; nausea; vomiting; hypertension; tachycardia; seizures; and anaphylaxis. These symptoms may last several days.
- *Interventions:* Support any airway, breathing, or circulation concerns first. Anticipate orders to treat the symptoms. These may include orders for ice pack to affected area, administration of analgesics or local anesthetics for pain, immobilization of the affected extremity to slow venom absorption, IV fluid bolus, antiemetics for vomiting, and/or antihistamines for swelling. The patient may need to be monitored for several hours to ensure there is no progression to a more severe reaction.

Notes: ____

STINGRAY STINGS

Stingrays are not typically aggressive creatures. They usually swim away if threatened. Most stings to humans are the result of a swimmer accidentally stepping on the back of the stingray.

- *Causes:* Sting from a stingray. If stepped on, the stingray instinctively whips its spikey venomous tail and may puncture the flesh of your patient (commonly on the leg). These spikes or spines may break off in the wound and continue to release venom.
- *Signs and symptoms:* May be local and/or systemic.
  - *Local:* Bleeding puncture wounds; lacerations; embedded spines; severe pain; muscle cramps; and swelling.
  - *Systemic:* Nausea; vomiting; diarrhea; headache; fever; chills; and hypotension.
- *Interventions:* Anticipate orders to place the affected area in warm water (about 113 °F) for about 6 to 90 minutes, taking care not to burn the patient. The warm water deactivates the venom and provides pain relief for the patient. The provider may also order local anesthetics, analgesics for pain, wound irrigation or debridement, prophylactic administration of antibiotics to prevent infection, and x-ray or ultrasound of the affected area to reveal any embedded barbs. The patient may require surgical exploration to remove all embedded barb fragments or spines. Prepare for possible OR admission. Preventive teaching should include teaching swimmers and divers to slide their feet across the ocean floor rather than stepping.

Notes: ____

Question: How long should the patient stung by a stingray soak their foot in hot water?
Answer: *Until the pain is relieved.*

SUMMARY

Environmental emergencies encompass a broad spectrum of injuries and illnesses. You may see one specific type of environmental emergency more than another, depending on your geographic area. Taking the time to learn about the most common environmental emergencies unique to your location is vital. If you are new to the area, ask your colleagues or preceptor what to expect. Be sure to note the duration and location of exposure for any type of environmental illnesses or injuries. No matter which environmental emergency arises, be sure to educate your patients on prevention and protection against future environmental dangers.

8

Fluid and Electrolyte Imbalances

As you already may know, **fluid and electrolyte balance is essential to maintaining homeostasis within the body.** It is important to understand the body's relationships between water and electrolytes. If not treated, interruptions to this balance can be fatal. Therefore, it is vital for the A&E nurse to recognize the most common manifestations of fluid and electrolyte imbalances and how to correct them. Oral replacements are preferred but sometimes intravenous (IV) correction is emergently necessary. The goal is to **slowly** restore fluid and electrolyte balance.

During this part of your orientation, locate and become familiar with:

- Doppler machine for pedal pulses
- Peritoneocentesis tray and fluid containers
- IV/intraosseous (IO) access equipment, policy, and procedure
- IV fluids: Normal saline (0.9%) or 3% if severe, Ringer's lactate, dextrose 5% in water (D5W), and dextrose 5% in 0.45% normal saline (D5$\frac{1}{2}$NS)
- Lab values: Basic or complete metabolic panel: sodium, potassium, calcium, phosphorus, and magnesium
- Medications to know: furosemide, potassium intravenously and by mouth, calcium chloride, calcium gluconate, sodium bicarbonate, magnesium sulfate, dextrose with IV regular insulin, sodium polystyrene sulfonate (Kayexalate), glucocorticoids, phosphate, calcitonin, and ethylenediaminetetraacetic acid

EDEMA

Edema occurs when plasma fluid shifts into the interstitial space. There are four different types of edema based on location and injury.

Pulmonary edema: Fluid shifts to the lungs.

- *Causes:* Left-sided congestive heart failure (CHF); chest trauma; anaphylactic shock; and septic shock.
- *Signs and symptoms:* Shortness of breath; jugular vein distention (JVD); and crackle breath sounds.
- *Interventions:* Anticipate orders to arrange for chest x-ray, provide oxygen, and give diuretics (furosemide).

Notes: ____

Ascites: Fluid shifts to the abdomen.

- *Causes:* Liver problems or abdominal trauma.
- *Signs and symptoms:* Abdominal swelling/edema. The patient may also have pedal edema.
- *Interventions:* Anticipate patient will receive a peritoneocentesis and other measures to correct underlying liver problems.

Notes: ____

Pedal edema: Fluid shifts to the lower extremities.

- *Causes:* Right-sided CHF; lower extremity trauma; peripheral vascular disease; cast applied too tightly; high-sodium diet; and lymphedema.
- *Signs and symptoms:* Feet swelling and edema.
- *Interventions:* Give diuretic as ordered (furosemide); assess pedal pulses; and document stage of edema.

Notes: ____

Severe burns: Fluid shifts to burned areas, causing localized edema.

- *Causes:* The body's natural response to a severe burn injury: swelling and fluid shift.
- *Signs and symptoms:* Localized edema to burn area.
- *Interventions:* Volume replacement. Patient is experiencing cellular dehydration.

Essential Facts

Most electrolyte imbalances effect your **neuromuscular system** in some form, including the heart muscle. Therefore, it is common to see muscle cramps, muscle twitching, abnormal reflexes, weakness, and cardiac dysrhythmias with nearly every electrolyte imbalance.

IV fluid memory trick:

- *Isotonic Fluids:* Stay where **I** put them, **I**nside the vessel.
- *HypOtonic Fluids:* Go **O**utside the vessel.
- *HypErtonic Fluids:* **E**nter the vessel.

Notes: ____

____

____

____

____

____

____

____

____

____

____

____

____

____

____

____

____

HYPONATREMIA

Hyponatremia means that sodium level in the blood is <135. **Remember that sodium follows water and chloride.** Where there is hyponatremia, there is also hypochloremia and dehydration.

- *Causes:* Syndrome of inappropriate antidiuretic hormone, medications (morphine sulfate, penicillin G, barbiturates, diuretics, mannitol, and oxytocin), and too much D5W; nausea, vomiting, and diarrhea; gastrointestinal suction; excessive sweating; Addison's disease; CHF; liver failure; renal failure; extracellular fluid loss (burns, peritonitis, and bowel obstruction); and CHF.
- *Signs and symptoms for Na <120:* Irritability; nausea and vomiting; fever; weakness; hypotension; headache; confusion; tachycardia; lethargy; abdominal cramps; and dry oral mucosa. Na levels <110: **seizures,** coma, and death.
- *Interventions:* Anticipate orders to correct fluid imbalances, intravenously administer normal saline 0.9% or 3% slowly if hyponatremia is severe, perform basic metabolic panel, and monitor closely. Goal is to change sodium levels at a rate ≤0.5 mEq/hr. Furosemide (Lasix) may be given to correct CHF.

Notes: ____

____

____

____

____

____

____

____

____

____

____

____

HYPERNATREMIA

Hypernatremia is a condition with sodium level >145. Again, because sodium follows chloride, hypernatremia = hyperchloremia. **Cellular dehydration is occurring.**

- *Causes:* Diabetes insipidus; poor fluid intake in hot weather; fever; infections; renal disease; diarrhea; excessive sweating; diaphoresis; hyperventilation; overly effective diuretics; Cushing's syndrome; and burns.
- *Signs and symptoms:* Anorexia; nausea; vomiting; agitation; thirst; oliguria; seizure; lethargy; coma; and muscle weakness/twitching.
- *Interventions:* Anticipate orders to obtain metabolic panel labs, give water by mouth, or to start an IV D5W or hypotonic saline. The goal is a **slow gradual correction to avoid cerebral edema and seizures**.

Notes: ____

____

____

____

____

____

____

____

____

____

____

____

____

____

____

HYPOKALEMIA

Hypokalemia is a condition with potassium level <3.5.

- *Causes:* Burns; gastrointestinal obstruction; acute alcoholism; diuretics; Cushing's syndrome (adrenal hyperactivity); dialysis; vomiting and diarrhea; **steroids**; uncontrolled diabetes mellitus; excessive sweating; or gastrointestinal suctioning.
- *Signs and symptoms:* Lethargy; fatigue; muscle weakness and decreased/absent deep tendon reflexes; tachycardia; parasthesia; paralysis; paralytic ileus; weak irregular pulse; tetany; orthostatic hypotension; and flatten/inverted T wave, **U waves,** and ST depression on an EKG. The U wave is additional wave after the T wave.
- *Interventions:* Anticipate orders to correct alkalosis (no sodium bicarbonate, no vomiting, no diarrhea, and no gastrointestinal suctioning), administer potassium by mouth or intravenously, perform basic metabolic panel, check magnesium, and give IV lactated Ringer's fluids.

Notes: ____

____

____

____

____

____

____

____

Essential Facts

- The correct infusion rate of an IV potassium drip is no faster than 20 mEq of potassium chloride per hour **on a pump**. Preferred dose is **10 mEq/hr via large-bore IV or central line.**
- If infused too quickly, potassium drip can cause **fatal arrhythmias** and phlebitis!

HYPERKALEMIA

Hyperkalemia is a condition in which the potassium level is >4.5.

- *Causes:* Renal failure; diabetes mellitus; crush injury; early burn stages; aldosterone deficiency; excessive potassium intake; potassium-sparing diuretics; angiotensin-converting enzyme (ACE) inhibitor medications; hyponatremia; and respiratory/metabolic acidosis.
- *Signs and symptoms:* **Muscle weakness**, cramps, and pain; dyspnea; **peaked T waves** and widened QRS on EKG; nausea, vomiting, and diarrhea; paresthesia; irritability; dysrhythmias; sinus bradycardia; first-degree heart block; ventricular fibrillation; and asystole.
- *Interventions:* Anticipate orders to monitor cardiac performance; restrict potassium intake (in food or medication); administer normal saline bolus intravenously; and give diuretics, Kayexalate by mouth or rectum, and possibly albuterol nebulizer. When IV medications are ordered, **give (IV) calcium chloride or calcium gluconate slow push over 5 to 10 minutes first to protect the heart**, then IV glucose (dextrose 50% injection [D50]), then IV regular insulin, and finally IV sodium bicarbonate. If given too fast, the calcium bolus can cause hypotension.

Figure 8.1 illustrates EKG changes during hypokalemia and hyperkalemia. You can see how potassium directly affects the heart.

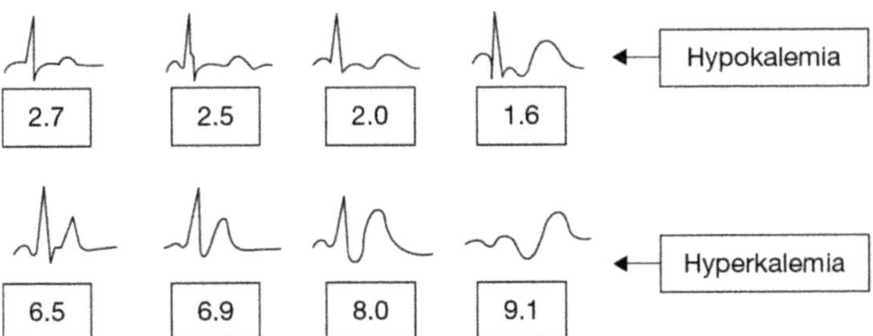

Figure 8.1 EKG changes in potassium imbalances.

Essential Facts

- It is normal to have a high potassium level with high blood sugar.
- As the blood sugar decreases with insulin treatment, the potassium will shift into the cell, and the serum potassium level will drop.

Notes: ____

____

____

____

____

____

____

____

____

____

____

____

____

____

____

____

____

____

____

____

____

____

HYPOCALCEMIA

Hypocalcemia is a condition in which the serum calcium level is <8.5 to 9 or an ionized calcium <4.5. It leads to increased **neuromuscular excitability**. Calcium counterbalances phosphate; therefore, hypocalcemia = hyperphosphatemia. Calcium follows magnesium; hypocalcemia = hypomagnesemia.

- *Causes:* Hypoparathyroidism; vitamin D deficiency; peritonitis; bone cancer; calcium channel blocker overdose; acute pancreatitis; burns; renal failure; sepsis; shock; citrate (anticoagulant used in blood transfusions); trauma; rhabdomyolysis; alcoholism; and malnutrition.
- *Signs and symptoms:* Just remember **CATS**: **C**onvulsions, **A**nxiety, **T**etany, and **S**pasms. Other symptoms include irritability; nausea, vomiting, and diarrhea; muscle cramps; muscle twitching; hyperactive deep tendon reflexes; numbness/tingling to toes, nose, fingers, lips, and earlobes; dysrhythmias (**prolonged QT intervals**); unconsciousness; and cardiac failure.
  - *Chvostek's sign:* Facial muscle spasms when facial nerve tapped anterior to external ear below the temporal bone.
  - *Trousseau's sign:* Hand/carpal spasms when pumping up blood pressure cuff above systolic pressure for 3 minutes.
- *Interventions:* Anticipate orders to obtain repeat serum calcium and protein levels; administer normal saline intravenously, monitor cardiac performance, document blood pressures; give **slow** IV calcium chloride or calcium gluconate bolus, and correct magnesium deficit.

Notes: ____

____

____

____

____

____

____

____

____

HYPERCALCEMIA

Hypercalcemia is a condition with calcium level >10.6. It leads to decreased neuromuscular excitability. Phosphate counterbalances calcium. Therefore, hypercalcemia = hypophosphatemia. Calcium follows magnesium; hypercalcemia = hypermagnesemia.

- *Causes:* Renal disease; hyperparathyroidism; too much vitamin D; drinking too much milk; pancreatitis; peptic ulcers; Addison's disease; thiazide diuretics; and prolonged immobilization.
- *Signs and symptoms:* Muscle weakness; decreased deep tendon reflexes; dehydration; nausea and vomiting; anorexia; constipation; ileus; kidney stones; polyuria; polydipsia; lethargy; headache; irritability; decreased level of consciousness; dysrhythmias (short QT interval); and cardiac arrest.
- *Interventions:* Anticipate orders to administer diuretics and 1 to 2 L of normal saline bolus intravenously, monitor cardiac rhythm, perform basic metabolic panel, measure magnesium level, measure intake and output, monitor for cardiac heart failure, and administer medications (glucocorticoids, diuretics, calcitonin, phosphate, or ethylenediaminetetraacetic acid).

Notes: ____

____

____

____

____

____

____

____

____

Essential Facts

To remember symptoms of hypercalcemia, just use the following rhyming words: moans, groans, bones, stones, and psych overtones.

HYPOMAGNESEMIA

Hypomagnesemia is a condition in which serum magnesium level is <1.5 mEq/L and can be commonly found in hospitalized patients. Magnesium follows calcium. Therefore, hypomagnesemia also results in hypocalcemia.

- *Causes:* May include malnutrition, alcoholism, cirrhosis, ulcerative colitis, diabetic ketoacidosis, diuretics, or renal disease.
- *Signs and symptoms:* Weakness; lethargy; hypotension; bradycardia or dysrhythmias (prolonged QT intervals, **torsades de pointes,** and ventricular fibrillation [V-fib]); increased deep tendon reflexes; nausea; vomiting; coma; and bradypnea and may lead to cardiac or pulmonary arrest.
- *Interventions:* Anticipate orders to administer by mouth or IV magnesium, apply cardiac monitor, monitor vital signs, obtain repeat serum magnesium levels, assess deep tendon reflexes, and monitor intake and output and magnesium levels. IV magnesium has multiple indications with various IV drip rates. Be sure to become familiar with the concentrations available to you; do not give IV magnesium too fast or your patient could go into cardiopulmonary arrest.

Notes: ____

____

____

____

Essential Facts

IV magnesium has many doses that vary according to indication:
- For cardiac arrest due to hypomagnesemia or torsades de pointes, give 1 to 2 g diluted in 10 mL of D5W IV/IO.
- For torsades de pointes with a pulse or acute myocardial infarction with hypomagnesemia, give 1 to 2 g diluted in 50 to 100 mL D5W over 5 to 60 minutes IV.
- For hypomagnesemia, give 1 g diluted in 50 mL D5W over 30 to 60 minutes IV.

HYPERMAGNESEMIA

Hypermagnesemia is a condition in which the serum magnesium level is >2.3 mEq/L.

- *Causes:* May include magnesium overdose, renal disease, or adrenocortical insufficiency.
- *Signs and symptoms:* Lethargy; nausea; headache; diminished or absent deep tendon reflexes; muscle weakness or paralysis; bradypnea or apnea; hypotension; hypocalcemia; EKG changes (atrioventricular blocks); and cardiac or respiratory arrest.
- *Interventions:* Anticipate orders to monitor cardiac rhythms, deep tendon reflexes, vital signs, and magnesium levels; to administer calcium gluconate or furosemide (Lasix) with saline diuresis. If severe, dialysis may be ordered.

Notes: ____

____

____

____

____

____

____

____

____

____

____

____

____

____

____

____

____

OVERHYDRATION

Overhydration is also known as "fluid overload."

- *Causes:* Drinking too much water or fluids; receiving too much IV fluid, long-term corticosteroid use, and overproduction of antidiuretic hormone; and medical conditions such as CHF and renal failure.
- *Signs and symptoms:* Pedal/pulmonary edema; nausea and vomiting; headache; anorexia; confusion; seizure; aphasia; or blurred vision.
- *Interventions:* Anticipate orders to restrict fluids, give diuretics, monitor and document intake and output, and document level of consciousness.

Notes: ____

____

____

____

____

____

____

____

____

____

____

____

____

____

____

____

____

DEHYDRATION

Dehydration is a lack of fluids.

- *Causes:* Inadequate fluid intake; diuretics; burns; third spacing (internal bleeding, crush injury); and vomiting or diarrhea. Fever and excessive sweating are not measurable but may result in excessive insensible fluid loss. Geriatrics and pediatrics are high-risk populations.
- *Signs and symptoms:* Confusion; disorientation; seizure; dry oral mucosa; dry skin; hyperthermia; weak rapid pulse; orthostatic hypotension; lethargy; fever; thirst; sunken fontanelles and eyes in infants; lack of tears in crying children; concentrated urine; tachypnea; tachycardia; and decreased urine output.
- *Interventions:* Anticipate orders to give fluids intravenously or by mouth, administer antipyretics for fever, perform basic metabolic panel and EKG, document mental status, check orthostatic vital signs, and measure intake and output.

Notes: ____

____

____

____

____

____

____

____

____

____

____

____

____

____

SUMMARY

Fluids and electrolytes play a key role in health and homeostasis. The kidneys act as the gatekeeper for most fluids and electrolytes. It is critical that A&E nurses understand this delicate balance, as a slight disturbance to this amazing balance can be fatal. Electrolytes typically affect the neuromuscular system. Make sure you learn the different lab values; you will need them every day in evaluating a wide variety of illnesses.

9

Gastrointestinal Emergencies

The gastrointestinal (GI) system is made up of several organs, including the stomach, liver, pancreas, gallbladder, and intestines. GI emergencies can be a very messy everyday A&E occurrence. Ruptured bowels, vomiting, diarrhea, constipation, enemas, you name it; you will see all types of GI problems in the A&E. Catching the projectile vomit in the basin is the real trick! After reviewing this chapter, you will be able to differentiate the types of GI emergencies and their causes, manifestations, and treatments. **For each patient, complete a full GI assessment and document thoroughly.**

During this part of your orientation, locate and become familiar with:

- Suction equipment
- Gastric lavage equipment and nasogastric tubes
- Hemoccult and gastroccult specimens
- Enemas
- Emergency endoscopy procedures
- Esophageal tamponade tubes
- Basins, Chux, and incontinence pads or liners
- Medications to know: GI cocktail, famotidine (Pepcid), pantoprazole (Protonix), promethazine (Phenergan), metoclopramide (Reglan), and ondansetron hydrochloride (Zofran)

Table 9.1

PQRST Abdominal Pain Assessment	
Component	**Description**
Provocation	What makes pain better or worse? Position?
Quality or character	Describe: burning, aching, sharp, dull, cramping, stabbing
Radiation, referral location	Where does pain radiate? Where does it start?
Severity	How severe is pain on scale of 0–10?
Time	When did is start and end? How long did is last?

NEVER UNDERESTIMATE ABDOMINAL PAIN

I once had a female patient come in by ambulance complaining of abdominal pain for 5 minutes. I thought it was a little silly to call an ambulance after just 5 minutes of pain. She was hollering, wailing, and carrying on so much that I could barely get a history. She was seen, assessed by a doctor, and x-rayed in about 15 minutes. Then she said her chest hurt. It turned out she not only had a ruptured bowel but also was having an acute myocardial infarction at the same time! Boy, we were shocked! So, although a patient may appear to be very dramatic, **never underestimate abdominal pain.**

Essential Facts

- A patient who has vomited 20 times in the past 8 hours is at risk for *metabolic alkalosis and hypokalemia* (see Chapter 8).
- After ingesting bleach, the patient has corrosive injury to the esophagus. Initial assessment and treatment should include *airway management.*
- Causes of ascites include *constrictive pericarditis, cirrhosis,* and *peritonitis.*
- *Sepsis* is the most common problem associated with colon trauma.

Question: The abdomen is assessed in which order?
Answer: *Inspection, auscultation, percussion, and palpation (look, listen, and feel).*

GASTRITIS

Gastritis is an inflammation of the stomach lining that can be an acute or chronic condition. Chronic gastritis can lead to ulcers and GI bleeding.

- *Causes:* Infection; stress; acute illness; gastroesophageal reflux disease (GERD); aspirin; nonsteroidal anti-inflammatory drugs (NSAIDs); alcohol; or food poisoning.
- *Signs and symptoms:* Nausea and vomiting; diarrhea; gastric mucosal bleeding; epigastric pain; malaise; anorexia; and loss of appetite.
- *Interventions:* Anticipate orders to administer fluids intravenously; arrange for abdominal x-ray; provide blood if blood loss is severe; prepare a complete blood count, *Helicobacter pylori* testing, amylase level, and lipase and basic metabolic panel; and administer medications (e.g., antacids, GI cocktail, histamine receptor antagonists, and antiemetics). Discharge teaching should include lifestyle modifications of six small meals daily, smoking cessation, and prescribed use of antacids.

Notes: ____

Essential Facts

A GI cocktail is made up of a liquid antacid and belladonna alkaloids/phenobarbital (Donnatal). (Adding 10 mL of viscous lidocaine makes it a super GI cocktail.)

Question: A 36-year-old male patient complains of burning epigastric pain 1 to 2 hours after eating, for 1 to 2 weeks. What is his diagnosis?

Answer: *Peptic ulcer disease.*

GASTROENTERITIS

Gastroenteritis is an inflammation of the stomach or small intestine. It is often the diagnosis when the patient says, "I think I have the stomach flu."

- *Causes:* Viruses; bacteria; parasites; toxins; or allergens. The most common viruses that cause gastroenteritis are **Norwalk virus and rotavirus.**
- *Signs and symptoms:* Nausea, vomiting, and diarrhea; hyperactive bowel sounds; abdominal pain or cramps; fever; dehydration; and hypovolemia in the very young or very old.
- *Interventions:* **Practice strict handwashing** and **contact precautions**; anticipate orders to provide fluids intravenously, prepare a basic metabolic panel and complete blood count, administer medications (antibiotics and antiparasitic agents), and provide patient education on a clear liquid and BRAT (bananas, rice, applesauce, and toast) diet.
  - Discharge teaching should include avoiding meat and dairy products, spicy foods, alcohol, greasy foods, and acidic foods.
  - Infants should not stop formula feeding for more than 24 hours.
  - Recovering from nausea and vomiting is a **gradual process**. The patient should have nothing by mouth (NPO) for an hour or so after vomiting. Then clear liquids should be introduced in small increments (ice chips) or one teaspoon every 5 minutes for the first 24 hours. Afterwards, the patient can advance to full liquids avoiding dairy. The next step is the BRAT diet; finally, the advanced diet as tolerated. Follow this process gradually or you will be cleaning up vomit!

Notes: ____

____

____

____

____

____

____

____

GASTROESOPHAGEAL REFLUX DISEASE

GERD is commonly called "acid reflux." It occurs when excess stomach acid travels up the esophagus, resulting in esophagitis.

- *Causes:* The malfunction of the esophageal sphincter and hiatal hernia are the major causes. Contributing factors are cigarette smoking; lying down after meals; stress; pregnancy; medications; and consuming alcohol, large meals, spicy or acidic food, and caffeine. Complications such as scar tissue, dysphagia, and esophageal strictures may result from repeated exposure to gastric content.
- *Signs and symptoms:* Upper midsternal burning pain and indigestion that worsens with lying down.
- *Interventions:* Anticipate orders for barium swallow, antacids, and GI cocktail. Educate the patient to avoid stress, fatty or fried foods, chocolate, alcohol, and overeating. The patient should drink plenty of water and avoid lying down for 3 hours after eating.

Notes: ____

____

____

____

____

____

____

____

____

____

____

____

INTESTINAL OBSTRUCTION

This is a potentially life-threatening condition resulting in the inability to move GI contents through the intestines. If untreated, mortality greatly increased. Your patient may present with severe pain and appear anxious. There are two types of obstructions: large bowel and small bowel. If you had to choose, you might prefer the early large-bowel obstruction, because nothing is coming out of either end. On the other hand, the patient with small-bowel obstruction will be continually vomiting and having diarrhea. You will need plenty of bedpans and emesis basins.

- *Causes:* Previous abdominal surgery, adhesions; hernia; strictures; foreign bodies; volvulus (twisting of bowel); intussusception; tumor; paralytic ileus; mesenteric infarction; and abdominal angina.
- *Signs and symptoms:* Fever; abdominal distention; nausea and vomiting; rapid onset of severe cramping abdominal pain; diffuse abdominal tenderness and rigidity; dehydration; weight loss or weight gain (due to fluid retention); high-pitched or absent bowel sounds; diaphoresis; weakness; restlessness; and constipation or recent diarrhea.
- *Interventions:* Anticipate orders to arrange for abdominal CT scan, ultrasound, or x-rays; monitor vital signs; give NPO; obtain complete blood count, amylase, alkaline phosphatase, lactic acid, and metabolic panel; administer fluids intravenously, antiemetics and analgesics; insert nasogastric tube for gastric decompression; administer antibiotic medications; and prepare for possible operating room (OR) admission.

Notes: ____

Tips for nasogastric tube insertion:
- Be nice when inserting a tube down a patient's *belly;* get a doctor's order to use lidocaine *jelly* to lubricate the tip.
- Apply oral anesthetic spray to the throat as ordered.
- Check placement initially by *auscultating stomach, confirming that the patient is able to speak,* and *checking gastric content.*
- To help the tube curve down the nasopharynx, curl the tip of the nasogastric tube around your finger first.

APPENDICITIS

Appendicitis is an inflammation and obstruction of the appendix. It typically occurs in males ages 10 to 19 but can happen to anyone. It affects 7% of the population. If untreated, it can become necrotic or perforate. If it ruptures, it could lead to peritonitis, sepsis, and then septic shock!

- *Causes:* Unknown, but may be attributed to infection, twisting, or obstruction of the appendix.
- *Signs and symptoms:* **Constant dull right lower-quadrant abdominal pain** (McBurney's point; see Figure 9.1); rebound tenderness; elevated white blood cell (WBC) count; nausea and vomiting; low-grade fever (usually after first 24 hours); and manifestations of peritonitis (fever, guarding, abdominal pain and distention, hypoactive bowel sounds, and diffuse rigidity). *With appendicitis, the pain typically precedes the vomiting. The patient is generally in so much pain that they vomit as a result of the pain.*
- *Interventions:* Anticipate orders to give patient NPO, analgesics, antibiotics, antiemetics, and fluids intravenously. Arrange for a complete blood count, metabolic panel, type and screen, an abdominal CT scan or ultrasound, and possible surgery.
  - A patient sent to surgery should have a completed preoperative checklist and be wearing only a gown. There should be *no body jewelry in unusual places, no hearing aids, no dentures, no hairpins, no socks, no underwear—just a patient gown.*

Notes: ____

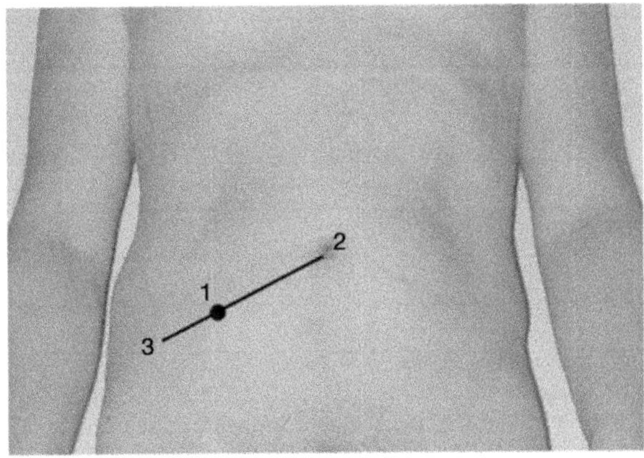

Figure 9.1 McBurney's point.

ESOPHAGEAL OBSTRUCTION

Esophageal obstruction, or food bolus, is a term for food or foreign bodies that get stuck or lodged in the esophagus. Meats such as steak, pork, and poultry can easily become lodged in the esophagus. This may be why some refer to esophageal obstruction as the "steakhouse syndrome."

- *Causes:* Ingestion of a foreign object or simply not chewing well before swallowing. Other conditions pose an increased risk for esophageal obstruction, such as esophageal cancer, eosinophilic esophagitis, nutcracker esophagus, peptic strictures, and Schatzki rings.
- *Signs and symptoms:* Foreign body sensation: "I have something stuck in my throat." The patient may also have acute dysphagia, chest pain, neck pain, pain with swallowing, regurgitation of food, and drooling.
- *Interventions:* Treat any airway concerns first. Anticipate orders to obtain x-rays of the chest and soft-tissue films of the neck, administer intravenous glucagon to relax esophageal smooth muscles, or prepare for endoscopy to retrieve the object. Patient discharge teaching should include chewing food thoroughly and use of dentures if applicable.

Notes: ____

____

____

____

____

____

____

____

____

____

____

____

ESOPHAGEAL VARICES (BLEEDING)

Esophageal varices are enlarged or varicosed veins located in the lower part of the esophagus.

I will never forget the night I first cared for a patient with bleeding esophageal varices. He was a man in his 40s, who came in via ambulance in full-fledged hypovolemic shock! His wife stated he was an alcoholic. He was as pale as the bed sheet beneath him, hypotensive, diaphoretic, tachycardic, semiconscious, and vomiting copious amounts of bright red blood. We had 3 units of O-negative blood rapidly infusing when the OR team arrived to perform an emergency endoscopic procedure right on the spot! The doctor finally was able to tie off the bleeding esophageal vessel. The patient was later admitted to the ICU and developed disseminated intravascular coagulation due to massive blood loss. At the time, I had never imagined one could lose so much blood from ruptured esophageal varices.

- *Causes:* Liver damage can lead to poor circulation through the portal vein, causing blood to back up into surrounding smaller vessels, such as esophageal veins. These fragile thin veins in the esophagus can then burst or rupture and bleed out into the esophagus. Other causes include thrombus, infection, and damage from liver cirrhosis.
- *Signs and symptoms:* Vomiting bright red blood, or dark and tarry stools. In severe cases, your patient may go into hemorrhagic/hypovolemic shock and require one-to-one monitoring.
- *Interventions:* Don necessary personal protective equipment (PPE) and treat any airway emergencies first. Anticipate orders to administer oxygen, beta-blockers such as propranolol, and medications to decrease portal vein pressure (octreotide, somatostatin, or vasopressin and nitroglycerin); insert large-bore intravenous access; monitor vital signs; assess and treat patient for any signs of hypovolemic shock; obtain type and crossmatch for possible blood transfusion; insert balloon tamponade tube; and prepare for endoscopy.

Notes: ____

____

____

____

____

CHOLECYSTITIS

Cholecystitis is an inflammation of the gallbladder.

- *Causes:* Gallstones; obstruction; or acute inflammation.
- *Signs and symptoms:* Right upper-quadrant abdominal pain radiating to back or right shoulder that becomes worse after eating fatty foods; low-grade fever; tachycardia; clay-colored stool; nausea and vomiting; anorexia; flatulence; possible jaundice; fat intolerance; and Murphy's sign.
- *Interventions:* Anticipate orders to obtain gallbladder ultrasound, complete blood count, liver enzymes, serum amylase, hepatobiliary iminodiacetic acid (HIDA) scan, and abdominal CT; give NPO; administer fluids intravenously; give medications (analgesics, antibiotics, sedatives for smooth muscle relaxation, and antiemetics for nausea and vomiting); and use nasogastric tube for gastric decompression. Arrange for possible surgical intervention.
  - *Morphine sulfate should be avoided.* It can cause gallbladder spasms.
  - **Murphy's sign** is an increased sharp right upper-quadrant abdominal pain that occurs during inspiration when palpating the patient's gallbladder and asking the patient to take a deep breath.
  - To palpate the gallbladder, press the fingers under the right anterior rib cage.

Notes: ____

____

____

____

____

____

____

____

____

____

GASTROINTESTINAL BLEEDING

GI bleeding can be classified as upper or lower. Patients with GI bleeding have a distinct odor. Once you have learned it, you can identify a patient with GI bleeding a mile away!

Upper Gastrointestinal Bleeding

- *Causes:* Peptic ulcer; stomach cancer; infection; esophageal varices; and trauma.
- *Signs and symptoms:* Weakness, hypotension, hypovolemic shock, nausea, and vomiting; bright red to coffee ground color emesis; and **black tarry stools (melena)** or dark red rectal bleeding.
- *Interventions:* Anticipate orders to apply pulse oximetry; give oxygen; begin cardiac monitoring; start an 18- or 16-gauge intravenous access; prepare a complete blood count—hemoglobin and hematocrit, metabolic panel, and coagulation studies; arrange for abdominal CT scan; insert nasogastric tube; document gastric content findings; assess guaiac gastric contents and stool; administer fluids intravenously; give histamine antagonists; test blood for type and crossmatch; and prepare for possible blood transfusion or endoscopy.

Lower Gastrointestinal Bleeding

- *Causes:* Internal or external hemorrhoids; constipation; polyps; colitis; diverticulitis; colon cancer; and irritable bowel syndrome.
- *Signs and symptoms:* **Bright red rectal bleeding (hematochezia)**.
- *Interventions:* Anticipate orders to open large-bore intravenous access, prepare a complete blood count and coagulation studies, arrange for abdominal CT scan, assess guaiac gastric contents and stool, administer fluids intravenously, test blood for type and crossmatch, reverse coagulopathies, and prepare for possible blood transfusion.

Notes: ____

____

____

____

- Ulcerative colitis and Crohn's disease are inflammatory disorders of the colon and rectal mucosal lining. They can cause diffuse rectal bleeding.
- Ingesting bismuth subsalicylate (Pepto-Bismol), iron, and charcoal results in dark/black stools similar to those seen in upper GI bleeding.

Question: Your patient arrives with a history of alcohol abuse and cirrhosis. He is vomiting copious amounts of bright red blood. Vital signs are as follows: blood pressure of 82/56, pulse of 144, respirations of 36, and temperature of 99.8 °F. What do you do first?

Answer: *Suction blood from the airway (remember airway, breathing, and circulation [ABCs] first).*

SUMMARY

GI emergencies are daily events in the A&E. You should now be able to differentiate the various types of GI emergencies. Treat ABCs first. Be sure to assess, reassess, and document abdominal assessments carefully (Table 9.1). Abdominal pain may involve a serious problem. Consider the cause of the patient's symptoms and manage pain in a timely manner.

10

Genitourinary Emergencies

Genitourinary emergencies are routinely seen and treated in the A&E. Most of the time, they are minor problems that can be treated with medications. **However, genitourinary problems such as testicular torsion can result in loss of the testicle(s) if untreated.** This chapter guides you through the genital and urinary problems commonly faced in the A&E. After reviewing this chapter, you will understand the causes, manifestations, and interventions for common genitourinary emergencies.

During this part of your orientation, locate and become familiar with:

- Different types of urinary catheters (indwelling, intermittent, coudé, condom, and external female)
- Bladder irrigation systems
- Urine specimen collection supplies
- Urinals
- Urine strainers
- **Oliguria:** urine output <500 mL/day
- **Anuria:** no urine output
- **Hematuria:** blood in urine
- **Dysuria:** painful urination
- **Nocturia:** up all night voiding
- **Pyuria:** infection (white blood cell counts [WBCs]) in the urine

URINARY TRACT INFECTION

This is a bacterial infection of the bladder and urethra.

- *Causes:* Because of their anatomy, urinary tract infections are more common in women than in men. Other contributing factors are holding your urine, not drinking enough water, intercourse, kidney stones, and pH imbalances.
- *Signs and symptoms:* Dysuria; hematuria; frequency; nocturia; urgency; cloudy urine; foul-smelling urine; fever; urinary retention; and abdominal/suprapubic pain.
- *Interventions:* Obtain clean-catch urine or catheterized urine if vaginal bleeding is present, administer antibiotic as ordered, encourage fluids such as cranberry juice and water, discourage caffeinated drinks, discourage bubble baths, encourage sitz baths, teach to wipe from front to back after toileting, and teach sexually active females to void and cleanse perineal area after intercourse. If administering urinary analgesia (phenazopyridine), indicate that it will turn the urine orange and permanently stain underwear.

Notes: ____

____

____

____

____

____

____

____

____

____

____

____

PYELONEPHRITIS

This is a bacterial infection of the kidney or renal pelvis.

- *Causes:* Pyelonephritis usually starts as a urinary tract infection in the urethra or bladder that travels all the way up to the kidneys.
- *Signs and symptoms:* Flank pain; painful urination (dysuria); hematuria (macro or micro); frequency; urgency; cloudy urine; foul-smelling urine; fever; chills; costovertebral tenderness, and nausea and vomiting (NV). Urinalysis may reveal elevated WBC counts, nitrates, elevated red blood cell counts, and bacteria.
  - *Chronic pyelonephritis* (renal failure): Urine output <30 mL/hr (oliguria); elevated blood urea nitrogen and creatinine; hypertension; rapid weight gain; and altered loss of consciousness.
- *Interventions:* Obtain clean-catch urine or catheterized urine if vaginal bleeding is present, urinalysis, urine culture, blood cultures, complete blood count (CBC), intravenous (IV) fluids, and antibiotic/antipyretics/antiemetics as ordered; encourage intake of fluids such as cranberry juice and water, discourage caffeinated drinks, discourage bubble baths, encourage sitz baths and bed rest, teach females to wipe from front to back after toileting, teach sexually active females to void and cleanse perineal area before and after intercourse, and prepare for possible admission.

Notes: ____

____

____

____

____

____

____

____

____

____

RENAL CALCULI

Renal calculi are stones of various sizes along the urinary tract that are commonly known as "kidney stones" (Figure 10.1). The pain that they cause is equal to that experienced during childbirth!

- *Causes:* Kidney stones are usually made of calcium or uric acid salt deposits, possibly resulting from urine that is too alkaline or too acidic.
- *Signs and symptoms:* **Severe flank pain radiating to the groin**; restlessness; diaphoresis; NV; urgency; frequency; dysuria; hematuria; oliguria; pallor; low-grade fever; and guarding.
- *Interventions:* Anticipate orders to obtain clean-catch or catheter urine if vaginal bleeding is present; start IV line; administer analgesics (IV ketorolac) and document effectiveness; administer antiemetic medications; instruct to strain all urine; and prepare for CT scan of abdomen/pelvis without contrast. Do not forget to send patient home with a urine strainer.

Notes: ____

____

____

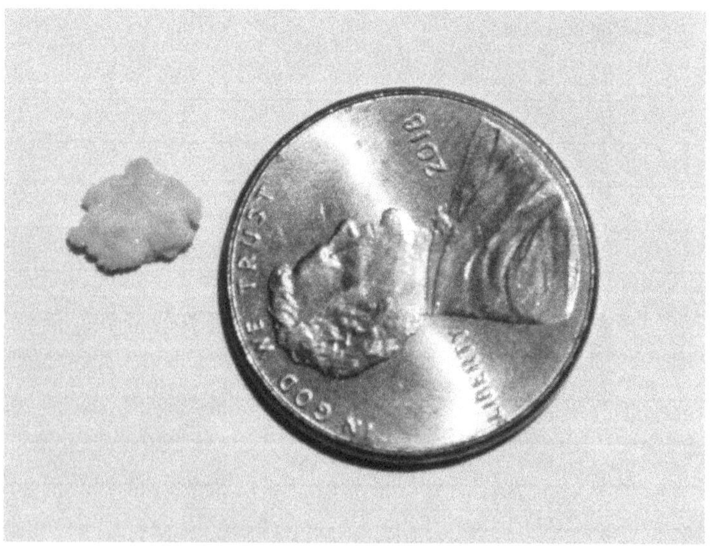

Figure 10.1 Renal calculi.

EPIDIDYMITIS

Epididymitis is an intrascrotal infection.

- *Causes:* Sexually transmitted diseases or urinary tract infections.
- *Signs and symptoms:* Penile discharge, bacteria in urinalysis, gradual scrotum **pain that is relieved with elevation**, fever, epididymis swelling, and chills.
- *Interventions:* Anticipate orders for ice pack to the scrotum, gonorrhea and chlamydia (G & C) culture, and antibiotics; instruct to abstain from sexual intercourse until follow-up repeat negative culture obtained.

Notes: ____

____

____

____

____

____

____

____

Essential Facts

When preparing ceftriaxone (Rocephin) intramuscular (IM) injection, 1% lidocaine may be used as a diluent to decrease discomfort. Caution lidocaine use in pediatric patients. Check for allergies to cephalosporins and lidocaine.

Question: A positive **Prehn sign** (pain relief with elevation of the effected testicle) is present in which condition? Epididymitis or testicular torsion?

Answer: *Epididymitis.*

TESTICULAR TORSION

This occurs when a testis spontaneously twists one or more times on the cord, leading to possible ischemia. The most common age group is 12 to 18 years old.

- *Causes:* It is not always known, but it can be attributed to an anatomic abnormality known as the "bell clapper deformity." This deformity allows the cords to twist more easily.
- *Signs and symptoms:* Acute, sudden, severe testicular pain radiating to groin or abdomen not relieved with testicle elevation; NV; and elevated/swollen/tender testes. **Absence** of the **cremasteric reflex** (elevation of the affected testis when aspect of inner thigh involved is gently stroked).
- *Interventions:* Anticipate orders for IV crystalloid fluids and analgesics, ice packs, and testicular ultrasound; prepare for manual reduction of the torsion or prepare for surgery as indicated.

Notes: ____

____

____

____

____

____

____

____

____

____

____

____

____

____

PENILE FRACTURE

Penile fracture is an acute rupture in the membrane (tunica albuginea) that surrounds the corpora cavernosa.

- *Causes:* Trauma or abrupt bending of the erect penis commonly associated with aggressive sexual intercourse or masturbation.
- *Signs and symptoms:* The patient may report hearing a cracking or popping sound upon injury, immediately followed by pain, flaccidity, hematoma, swelling, deformity, and dark bruising of the penis. Other symptoms may include hematuria, blood noted at the urethral meatus, and inability to void.
- *Interventions:* Anticipate orders to administer pain medications, insert IV access, obtain urinalysis if possible, contact emergent consulting urologist, and give patient nothing by mouth and *no* **urethral catheterizations**. Prepare for retrograde urethrogram and surgical intervention with transfer to the operating room.

Notes: ____

____

____

____

____

____

____

____

____

____

____

____

____

URINARY RETENTION

Urinary retention (ischuria) is the inability to void or to fully empty the bladder.

- *Causes:* Enlarged prostate, constipation, infection, nerve dysfunction, urethral obstruction or strictures, kidney stones, blood clots, and some medications such as opioids, amphetamines, anticholinergics, antidepressants, and cyclooxygenase-2 (COX-2) inhibitor medications.
- *Signs and symptoms:* Unable to void or "only a little comes out"; bladder "feels full" or is distended; lower mid-abdominal pain; and patient may appear anxious.
- *Interventions:* To properly treat urinary retention, one must first find the cause by obtaining an accurate urologic history and assessment. Anticipate orders to obtain urology consult and insert Foley catheter. If resistance is met upon Foley catheter insertion, do not force; reattempt with a smaller or specialty Foley catheter per order. Once inserted, the patient typically finds instant relief. To avoid bladder spasms, clamp the Foley after the first 1,000 mL empties into the Foley bag. If blood clots are present, bladder irrigation system may be ordered.

Notes: ____

____

____

____

____

____

____

____

____

____

____

GENITAL WARTS

Genital warts (condylomata acuminate) is a viral sexually transmitted infection. The virus responsible is the human papilloma virus (HPV). It is estimated that about 50% of sexually active males and females will acquire HPV in their lifetime.

- *Causes:* Sexual contact with an infected partner.
- *Signs and symptoms:* Painless single or multipapular-type rash in various shapes such as plaque or cauliflower-like appearance to the genital areas. Areas affected may include perianal, vulva, penis, perineum, and cervix. The oral pharynx or larynx may also be affected. Warts may spontaneously increase or decrease without treatment.
- *Interventions:* Because it is a viral infection, there is no cure. Treatments may include laser therapy, surgical excision, and/or cryotherapy. The treatment goal is to remove symptomatic warts to induce more "wart-free" periods. Although there is no cure, we can educate our patients on prevention. The Gardasil vaccine is now available to prevent cervical cancer and other diseases associated with HPV.

Notes: ____

____

____

____

____

____

____

____

____

____

____

____

PRIAPISM

Priapism is a prolonged painful penile erection lasting longer than 4 to 6 hours.

- *Common causes:* Spinal cord injury, leukemia, sickle cell disease, psychotropic drugs, multiple sclerosis, prolonged sexual stimulation, penile tumor, urethral tumor, anticoagulant therapy, and impotence treatments.
- *Signs and symptoms:* Prolonged painful penile erection for more than 4 to 6 hours.
- *Treatments:* Anticipate treatment of underlying causes by provider that may include observation of patient, ice packs, penile or groin pressure, intracavernous injections (with drugs such as epinephrine, norepinephrine, and ephedrine), needle aspiration, or surgery.

Notes: ____

____

____

____

____

____

____

____

____

____

____

____

Question: How do you treat a 19-year-old male who arrives at the A&E stating that his penis is stuck in his pants zipper?

Answer: *Cut it off: not the penis, the zipper! Control bleeding and provide ice packs.*

SUMMARY

Although most genitourinary emergencies can be treated with medications, some require immediate interventions. Remember that renal infections, obstructions, or poor perfusion can lead to renal failure; early intervention is key. Document your urine and genital assessments. Maintain and respect patient privacy; provide a chaperone when necessary. You should now understand some of the most frequent problems that bring patients to the A&E and how to treat them promptly and effectively.

11

Geriatric Emergencies

As the baby boomer generation ages, we are encountering an even higher volume of A&E patients. **The normal physiologic changes of the aging process leave patients more vulnerable to illness, injuries, and complications.** Several important body systems also slow down. Many geriatric patients have decreased renal function, decreased circulation, thinner skin, weaker bones, less muscle mass, decreased hearing, decreased gastric motility, brain atrophy, and visual impairments. It is always important to take these age-related changes into consideration when caring for older patients. As you review this chapter, you will learn some of the most common geriatric emergencies and how to handle them.

During this part of your orientation, locate and become familiar with:

- Assistive walking devices (e.g., canes and walkers)
- Adult protective services and social services
- Facility policy for reporting elder abuse
- Denture containers
- Fall risk assessments and precautions

SENSATORY CHANGES

- Touch—increase in threshold for touch, vibration, heat, and cold.
- Taste—taste buds decrease.
- Smell—little evidence that sense of smell diminishes with age.
- Hearing—severe changes to the structure of the inner ear, producing deficits in both hearing and equilibrium.
- Sight—decreased lens capsule elasticity, amplitude of accommodation, and shape and tone of ciliary body.

Essential Facts

Normal physiologic changes leave older patients more vulnerable to illness, injuries, and complications. Geriatric patients may have **decreased renal function**, decreased circulation, thinner skin, weaker bones, decreased hearing, decreased gastric motility, and visual impairments.

Question: Which lab levels naturally increase with age?
Answer: *Blood urea nitrogen and creatinine levels*

Notes: ____

____

____

____

____

____

____

____

____

____

____

ELDER ABUSE

Elder abuse can take several different forms, including physical, sexual, financial, and psychological; it can also include neglect. Abuse is physical harm, pain, or mental anguish; neglect is the failure to provide services or goods needed to prevent physical harm and mental anguish. Elder abuse is an international problem that can be difficult to detect. Females are more commonly abused than males. **You must report all suspected elder abuse!**

- *Causes:* Not always known. Elder abuse can occur in any socioeconomic group. Lack of resources and stressed or burned-out caregivers can contribute to the problem.
- *Signs and symptoms:* Conflicting stories describing how an injury occurred; patient not given an opportunity to speak; time lapse between injury and presentation to the A&E; disinterested caregiver; history of similar injuries; hand marks; bite marks; multiple bruises; multiple fractures in various healing stages; altered ambulation from sexual assault; malnourishment; dehydration; poor hygiene; withdrawal; and agitation.
- *Interventions:* Treat injuries and illness; *accurately document* and photograph injuries or neglect per policy; ascertain whether report needs to be filed; notify social services as soon as possible; obtain supportive services through community referrals; consider hospitalization to ensure patient safety; and refer to adult protective services.

Notes: ____

____

____

____

____

____

____

____

____

____

FALLS

Falls are the leading cause of hospital admissions and injury-related death in the geriatric population. Complications often include soft-tissue injuries, hip fractures, Colles' fracture (wrist), subdural hematoma, and hot-water burns from falls in the bathtub. First, **assess the reason for the fall**. Were there any symptoms prior to the fall (e.g., dizziness, chest pain, and loss of consciousness)? What was the activity during the fall? The location? Are there any witnesses? Any history of falls or alcohol intake? Finally, assess whether the patient fell at ground level. If not, how many feet did the patient fall?

- *Causes:* Can be attributed to impaired vision, sensation, neuro-circulatory system, gait, and balance.
- *Signs and symptoms:* Depend on the fall and injuries.
- *Interventions:* Give nothing by mouth; consider cervical injury and immobilization (rest, ice, splint, and elevate injury); clean and apply sterile dressing to wounds; assess pain; administer pain medications as ordered; arrange neurologic exams; monitor extremity movement; and check circulation. Prepare for diagnostic studies. Educate patient and family on fall prevention.

Notes: ____

____

____

____

____

____

____

____

____

____

____

____

____

____

SYNCOPE

Syncope is transient loss of consciousness with a spontaneous recovery.

- *Causes:* Identifying the cause may prove to be more valuable than treating the sustained injuries. Assess patient's activity just before the syncopal event.
  - Temporary, abrupt decrease in cardiac output due to aortic stenosis, mitral valve disease, cardiomyopathy, dysrhythmias, and sick sinus syndrome.
  - Volume depletion due to hemorrhage/anemia, diuresis, dehydration, and third-space fluid shift.
  - Hypersensitive carotid sinus due to neck turning, constrictive collars, and drugs (digitalis, propranolol hydrochloride, and alpha-methyldopa).
  - Vasovagal response with hypotension due to cough, defecation, or urination.
  - Hypoglycemia or hypoxia.
- *Signs and symptoms:* Dizziness; chest pain; dyspnea; weakness; confusion; loss of consciousness; witnesses to the fall; and previous history.
- *Interventions:* Anticipate orders to obtain serum glucose and complete basic metabolic panel; administer oxygen through nasal cannula; check pulse oxygen; perform EKG and CT scan.
  - If due to adult hypoglycemia, treat intravenously with dextrose 50% injection (D50; 1 amp) or give oral or intramuscular injection of glucose. Then feed patient once they are alert and oriented to person, place, and time.

Notes: ____

____

____

____

____

Question: What is the "classic" symptom of acute myocardial infarction in a geriatric patient 85 years of age or older?

Answer: *Shortness of breath may typically be seen instead of chest pain.*

DEHYDRATION

Dehydration is a lack of required serum fluid levels. Older adults are more prone to dehydration because of normal physiologic changes that occur with aging.

- *Causes:* Altered sense of thirst; decrease in total body fluid; decreased kidney function; and decreased effectiveness of antidiuretic hormone, which helps conserve water.
- *Signs and symptoms:* Confusion; seizure; dry oral mucosa; dry skin; sunken eyes; lethargy; headache; constipation; hyperthermia; weak rapid pulse; orthostatic hypotension; altered respiration; concentrated urine; and decreased urine output.
- *Interventions:* Anticipate orders to administer fluids intravenously or by mouth, assess mental status, check vital signs, and measure intake and output. Diagnostic studies may include metabolic panel, hematocrit, blood urea nitrogen, and complete blood count (CBC).

Notes: ____

____

____

____

____

____

____

____

____

____

____

____

____

____

____

DEMENTIA

Also known as "major neurocognitive disorder," dementia is commonly mistaken for normal age-related cognitive changes. However, with dementia, the onset is more severe with an abrupt onset.

- *Causes:* Not always known, but may be attributed to electrolyte imbalance, dehydration, infection, and stroke. This assessment requires input from caregivers to determine the patient's normal cognitive baseline.
- *Signs and symptoms:* Alert with impaired orientation; impaired recent memory; impoverished thinking; difficulty finding words; confused speech; and poor sleep.
- *Interventions:* Provide a safe environment; put bed in low, locked position; monitor patient closely (place close to nurses' station); and assess for any new causes of confusion. Anticipate orders for intravenous (IV) access, IV fluids, CBC with differential, metabolic panel, urinalysis, toxicology screen, chest x-ray, and head CT, and if possible, have family or sitter available at the bedside to redirect or reorient patient.
  - A common cause of confusion in older adults is *pneumonia* or *urinary tract infection.*

Notes: ____

____

____

____

____

____

____

____

____

____

____

____

____

ALZHEIMER'S DISEASE

Alzheimer's disease affects one in eight people older than 65 years of age. It is a chronic, progressive, irreversible, degenerative dementia that has no preventive measures or cure.

- *Causes:* Unknown with focus studies on loss of synapses in the brain.
- *Signs and symptoms:* Forgetfulness; memory loss; paranoia; delusions; irritability; depression; aphasia; apraxia; and history of progressive deteriorating mental functioning.
- *Interventions:* Prevent patient from injuring self or others; provide supervised safe environment with minimal stimulation; give short explanations and simple instructions; involve supportive services (social services); and provide health care resources and community referrals.

Notes: ____

____

____

____

____

____

____

____

____

____

____

____

____

____

____

____

____

____

PNEUMONIA

Pneumonia is a bacterial, viral, or fungal infection below the bronchi resulting in inflammation of lung parenchyma.

- *Causes:* Bacterial, viral, or fungal lung infection. Contributing factors include a weak immune system; general debilitated condition; decreased mobility; chronic cardiac disease; chronic pulmonary disease; **weak cough reflex**; decreased lung capacity; aspiration; late diagnosis; and diabetes.
- *Signs and symptoms:* **Confusion**; change in normal activity; anorexia; tachypnea; dyspnea; fever or subnormal temperature; dehydration; productive or nonproductive cough; chills; weakness; chest pain; nausea and vomiting; abdominal distention; diaphoresis; cyanosis; and diminished lung sounds or crackles.
- *Interventions:* Anticipate orders for chest x-ray, CBC, blood cultures, and arterial blood gases. Monitor and document work of breathing. Start IV access, maintain bed rest, and give fluids intravenously; pulse oximeter monitoring, along with oxygen and antibiotics as ordered.

Notes: ____

____

____

____

____

____

____

____

____

____

____

____

UROSEPSIS

Urosepsis is an infection caused by urinary tract infection that is more common in women than in men. In general, urinary infections are the most common bacterial infections in older adults. Urosepsis may lead to septic shock.

- *Causes:* Predisposing factors include an indwelling catheter and kidney stones.
- *Signs and symptoms:* Confusion; lethargy; altered mental status; tachycardia; tachypnea; fever or subnormal temperature; urinary frequency; urinary urgency; incontinence; nausea and vomiting; abdominal tenderness; and hypotension.
- *Interventions:* Anticipate orders to obtain urinalysis, administer fluids and antibiotics intravenously, and monitor urinary output. Prepare for possible admission.

Notes: ____

____

____

____

____

____

____

____

____

____

____

____

____

Question: What are the common causes associated with acute onset of altered mental status in older adult patients?
Answer: *Urosepsis and pneumonia.*

SUMMARY

You now have a better understanding of the diseases most commonly associated with older adults in the A&E. Age-related physiologic changes in older adults will affect their condition and can lead to complications. Be sure to assess and document these patients carefully. Obtain histories from them and their caregivers, when available. Caring for older adults can be a blessing. Often, they are kinder and more appreciative than younger patients.

12

Hematologic Emergencies

Some hematologic emergencies, such as anemia, sickle cell anemia, and hemophilia, are commonly seen in the A&E, while others, such as leukemia and lymphoma, are rarer. Regardless, an A&E nurse should be able to help identify and anticipate appropriate interventions. Remember to treat pain according to the patient's report. Just because you cannot see the pain does not mean it is not there. For example, a patient with sickle cell pain may play a game on their phone to distract from the pain. Document both subjective and objective data. Take the time to review your hospital's blood transfusion procedure with your preceptor; often, your colleagues in the blood bank department can serve as an excellent resource.

During this part of your orientation, locate and become familiar with:

- Blood transfusion supplies: blood tubing, forms and documentation, and hospital protocol
- Warming devices
- Neutropenic precautions
- Medications to know: morphine, hydromorphone (Dilaudid), ketorolac (Toradol), diphenhydramine (Benadryl), ondansetron (Zofran), promethazine (Phenergan), and factor VIII and IX replacement therapy

ANEMIA

Anemia, simply put, is a lack of oxygen-carrying red blood cells (RBCs) or hemoglobin. It can be mild or severe, acute or chronic. It is characterized by a low hemoglobin and hematocrit (H & H) level. In men, the normal hemoglobin level is <13.5% and the hematocrit level is <39 g/dL. In women, the normal hemoglobin level is <12% and the hematocrit is <36 g/dL.

- *Causes:* Blood loss due to trauma or gastrointestinal (GI) bleeding, destruction of RBCs, or inadequate RBC production. Common types of anemia include iron deficiency, vitamin deficiency, aplastic, hemolytic, sickle cell, thalassemia, and malarial. In addition, chronic inflammatory diseases, such as cancer, HIV, kidney disease, and Crohn's disease, and certain toxins or venoms can interfere with RBC production. It is not uncommon for patients older than 65 to have chronic mild anemia.
- *Signs and symptoms:* Weakness; fatigue; dizziness; headache; pallor; dyspnea; dysrhythmias; chest pain; and cool extremities.
- *Interventions:* Assess and treat underlying causes based on type of anemia. Anticipate orders to provide oxygen, control and reassess any hemorrhaging, establish large-bore intravenous (IV) access, monitor vital signs, monitor oximetry or waveform capnography, apply warming measure, and avoid nonsteroidal anti-inflammatory drugs (NSAIDs) if cause is bleeding. Anticipate orders to collect a complete blood count (CBC) with differential, coagulation studies, and type and crossmatch. Prepare for possible blood transfusion.

Notes: ____

____

____

Essential Facts

Quickly determine pallor regardless of skin type by assessing the palms of the patient's hands in addition to the inside lower eyelids and oral mucosa. Document a thorough circulatory assessment, including vital signs, capnometry, oximetry, color, temperature, and capillary refill of extremities before and after interventions to determine effectiveness.

SICKLE CELL ANEMIA

Sickle cell anemia is an inherited hemolytic form of anemia. The RBCs contain too much hemoglobin S, causing the RBC to take on a sickle or crescent-like shape instead of a normal tubular or jelly doughnut-like shape. Sickle-shaped blood cells tend to clump together in smaller or constricted vessels causing blockage or vaso-occlusive crisis (VOC). Similar to an acute myocardial infarction (AMI), the vessel obstruction can lead to poor tissue perfusion and eventually necrosis of surrounding tissue. Acute complications may include bacterial sepsis/meningitis, stroke, pulmonary embolism, acute chest syndrome (ACS), VOC, aplastic crisis, splenic sequestration, priapism, and papillary necrosis with hematuria. Chronic complications include anemia, jaundice, splenomegaly, functional asplenia, cardiomegaly, cholelithiasis, restrictive lung disease, avascular necrosis, pulmonary hypertension, renal failure, and retinal occlusion resulting in blindness.

- *Causes:* Inheriting two sickle cell genes from one's parents. According to the Centers for Disease Control and Prevention (CDC), sickle cell anemia affects millions of people around the world. Primarily it affects Black or African American patients, but is also found in Hispanic, Arabic, Indian, and Mediterranean patients. Although it is extremely risky, stem cell or bone marrow transplants offer a possible hope for a future cure.
- *Signs and symptoms:* Typically, patients present with **pain** but may also present with weakness, fatigue, dizziness, headache, pallor, dyspnea, dysrhythmias, chest pain, joint pain, delayed growth, fever, infections, and swollen or cool extremities.
- *Interventions:* Apply warming measures, pulse oximetry or waveform capnography, cardiac monitor, and supplemental oxygen if pulse oximetry reading is <92% to 94%. Anticipate orders for frequent vital signs, IV access, high-dose IV or subcutaneous opioids, analgesics, antiemetics, NSAIDs, and diphenhydramine (Benadryl). If patient is hypovolemic, isotonic crystalloid or hypotonic IV fluids may be ordered. It is recommended that analgesics be administered within 30 to 60 minutes of arrival. Blood transfusions may be ordered if the patient is in critical condition. Diagnostic tests may include CBC with differential, metabolic panel, reticulocyte count, and liver function test. Most sickle cell patients manage their disease proactively with their hematologists or primary care physicians. However, there will be a few who routinely use the A&E to

manage their care. A hospital or A&E social worker may be able to assist connecting the patient with better community sickle cell resources and follow-up care upon discharge. Discharge education should include follow-up and routine care with a hematologist; staying well hydrated; limiting exposure to cold and high altitudes; plenty of rest and exercise; warm, moist heat to reduce pain/swelling; genetic testing; and symptoms of ACS because it is a leading cause of death.

- *Serious Complications*:
  - **ACS: Dyspnea**, productive cough, hemoptysis, **chest pain**, and hypoxia are signs of **ACS**. Early recognition and interventions are vital to avoid respiratory failure and death.
  - **VOC:** Sickle cells clump together obstructing blood vessels leading to edema, tissue ischemia, severe pain, tissue necrosis, and organ dysfunction.

Notes: ____

____

____

Essential Facts

Patients with pain related to sickle cell disease are considered high risk according to the Emergency Severity Index (ESI). The suggested ESI level is 2 or high risk priority.

True or False: Diagnostic tests can be used to validate the pain in a sickle cell patient.
Answer: *False, patient report of severity should guide management of pain.*

Question: Decades ago, sickle cell anemia was considered a childhood illness as many did not survive to see adulthood. Today, the average life expectancy is
A. 30
B. 40
C. 50
D. 60
Answer: *B is correct.*

DISSEMINATED INTRAVASCULAR COAGULATION

Disseminated intravascular coagulation (DIC) typically results from a primary complication that triggers a massive coagulation pathway in the body. As a result, thrombocytopenia, fibrinolysis, and thrombosis may occur leading to systemic bleeding and micro-coagulation.

- *Causes:* A primary infection or inflammatory process; trauma; burns; shock; obstetric emergencies; sepsis; snake bite; heat stroke; or cancer.
- *Signs and symptoms:* Uncontrolled bleeding; petechial rash; purpura rash; oozing blood from venipuncture sites; hypoxia; and organ necrosis.
- *Interventions:* Anticipate orders to control any external hemorrhage; give oxygen; treat primary causes; obtain multiple large-bore IV accesses; and administer fresh frozen plasma (FFP), platelets, and cryoprecipitate with fibrinogen as ordered.

Notes: ____

____

____

____

____

____

____

____

____

____

____

____

____

____

HEMOPHILIA

Hemophilia is a rare congenital bleeding disorder related to poor clotting. It occurs primarily in males.

- *Causes:* Genetic defect of clotting factor VIII (type A) or clotting factor IX (type B or Christmas disease). This particular genetic defect was first reported in 1952 in a patient named Stephen Christmas. It is passed down from mother to son. Genetic researchers continue to search for a cure.
- *Signs and symptoms:* Excessive internal or external bleeding; bruising; prolonged nasal bleeding; hematuria; tarry stools; coffee-ground emesis; warm painful joint swelling; or signs of increased cranial pressure (ICP) if bleeding is present in the brain.
- *Interventions:* Triage a high-risk priority patient (ESI level 2). Anticipate orders to obtain IV access and immediate administration of clotting factor VIII or IX replacement IV as indicated. Other orders may include desmopressin acetate (DDAVP) administration for minor bleeding and joint elevation; ice; and immobilization, hematologist consult, and topical thrombin for nose bleeds. Diagnostic tests should not delay IV clotting factor replacement but may include CTs, x-rays, CBC, prothrombin time (PT), partial thromboplastin time (PTT), and factor levels. Most parents are a helpful resource as their children receive infusions weekly or routinely as preventative maintenance; they may even carry their own factor replacement with them to the A&E.

Notes: ____

____

____

Essential Facts

Intramuscular (IM) injections and repeated venipunctures in a hemophiliac patient should be avoided, as they may result in large painful hematomas. When obtaining labs and IV access, consider the following:

- utilizing an experienced IV therapist
- tying the tourniquet loosely to avoid bruising
- using smaller gauge needle if patient is hemodynamically stable
- applying direct pressure for 3 to 5 minutes afterward

LEUKEMIA

Leukemia is a cancer of the blood, blood-producing organs, and bone marrow.

- *Causes:* Damaged DNA or mutated bone marrow cells lead to an overproduction of blast cells, the precursors to white blood cells (WBCs). These cancerous blast cells never develop into healthy blood cells affecting platelet, RBC, and WBC production. There are several types of leukemia. The cause of this mutation is unknown but risk factors may include previous exposure to chemotherapy or radiation, chemical exposures such as benzene, family history of leukemia, smoking, and Down syndrome.
- *Signs and symptoms:* May include bruising; pallor; dyspnea; petechial or purpura rash; epistaxis; weakness; loss of appetite; weight loss; fever; frequent opportunistic infections; joint pain; swollen lymph nodes; splenomegaly; and hepatomegaly.
- *Interventions:* Anticipate orders to obtain CBC with differential, coagulation studies, chemistry, CT, x-rays, lumbar puncture (LP), and large-bore IV access. Possible blood transfusion, antibiotics, hematologist or oncologist consult, and neutropenic precautions may also be ordered. Definitive diagnosis may be made following a bone marrow biopsy.

Notes: ____

____

____

____

____

Question: Which nursing action is of greatest priority for a patient with bone pain related to leukemia?
A. Administer pain medication.
B. Place patient in a private room.
C. Administer oxygen.
D. Discuss advance directives.
Answer: *B is correct.*

Leukemia patients are highly susceptible to infection; a nosocomial infection could prove deadly. Place patient on reverse isolation upon arrival.

LYMPHOMA

Lymphoma is a rare cancer of the lymphatic system.

- *Causes:* Unknown but risk factors may include certain types of chemical, viral, or bacterial exposures; can be further classified into Hodgkin's and non-Hodgkin's lymphoma. Patients may present to the A&E with obstructions and immunosuppression complications.
- *Signs and symptoms:* **Painless swollen lymph nodes**; abdominal pain or swelling; chest pain; cough; dyspnea; fatigue; fever; night sweats; and weight loss. Complications may include swelling of upper airway, hypercalcemia, pericardial effusion with tamponade, spinal cord syndrome, DIC, and superior vena cava syndrome.
- *Interventions:* Treat airway, breathing, and circulation (ABCs) first, and anticipate orders for CBC with differential, coagulation studies, erythrocyte sedimentation rate, liver functions, blood urea nitrogen (BUN), creatinine, LP if neurologic system is affected, x-rays, CTs or MRIs of affected areas, and neutropenic precautions if patient is receiving chemotherapy or radiation. An endocrine or oncologist referral may be obtained to confirm diagnosis with lymph node or bone marrow biopsy.

Notes: ____

SUMMARY

Due to advances in treatment options, patients today are surviving and living longer with hematologic diseases. Anemia, sickle cell crisis, and hemophilia are more commonly seen in the A&E than other hematologic emergencies. Sickle cell pain interventions should be initiated ideally within 30 to 60 minutes of arrival. Be sure to review your hospital's process for type and crossmatch and blood transfusions. Ensure proper documents are completed such as blood consent, blood request, and transfusion assessments.

13

Infectious Disease Emergencies

Infectious diseases are common emergencies that must not be taken lightly. Usually, it is the triage nurse who is first exposed to an unknown case of tuberculosis, meningitis, or new viral pandemic. Most patients don't know what is wrong with them when they come to the A&E. Your facility should have a travel and triage screening process to help identify these cases to alert the staff of such infectious diseases and risks. The travel and triage screening may include questions about fever, cough, and travel within the past 21 days to a country or place of concern for pandemics, epidemics, or signs and symptoms of a transmissible disease. If the triage or travel screening is positive, you must follow your facility's protocol; this usually requires transmission-based precautions. The best advice I can give you is to assess your patients **carefully.** If you suspect that a patient may have any of the transmissible diseases, **isolate them, then consult** to verify, and **wash your hands, wash your hands, wash your hands!** Most A&E nurses frequently catch more colds and flus in their first year, so be careful. This chapter educates you on the different types of infectious diseases and how to handle them.

During this part of your orientation, locate and become familiar with:

- Wound cultures
- Lumbar puncture supplies, specimens, and procedures
- Contact, respiratory, airborne, and reverse isolation policies
- Personal protective equipment
- Incision and drainage supplies
- Triage screening for infectious diseases (HIV, tuberculosis [TB], fever, cough, travel in the past 21 days)
- Policy for reporting diseases to infection control personnel

Always practice universal/standard precautions.

CLOSTRIDIUM DIFFICILE INFECTION

Clostridium difficile (C. diff) is a bacterial infection of the colon that affects more than half a million people annually and is becoming more difficult to treat. It is spread via contaminated feces or unwashed hands and ingestion. Its spores can survive for weeks to months.

- *Causes:* Exposure to spore-producing *C. diff* bacteria or recent use of antibiotics. In the past, old age and exposure in healthcare facilities posed increased risks. Today, community-acquired *C. diff* is becoming more prevalent.
- *Signs and symptoms:* Severe frequent liquid diarrhea, abdominal pain and cramping, nausea, fever, and abdominal distention. Diarrhea containing *C. diff* has a distinct foul odor; many experienced nurses can walk into a room and identify *C. diff* based solely on odor. I have known patients suffering from *C. diff* who constantly leaked liquid diarrhea. After continual changing of disposable pads, diapers, and bed linen, a rectal tube was ordered.
- *Interventions:* Place the patient on contact-enteric precautions and implement strict handwashing with soap and water. Anticipate orders for intravenous (IV) fluids, antibiotics, complete blood count with differential, basic metabolic panel, and stool culture. Patients with mild infection may be treated with probiotics; patients with severe infection may require antibiotics and admission. Order and send stool specimens as soon as possible to help quickly diagnose so that treatment and management can begin. Remember to use bleach wipes to clean the patient's rooms. Do not remove isolation signage and supplies until environmental personnel have cleaned the room and made it ready for use.

Notes: ____

____

____

____

MENINGITIS

Meningitis is a bacterial, viral, or fungal infection of the meninges, which are membrane coverings of the brain. Bacterial meningitis is more serious and can lead to septic shock.

- *Causes:* It usually starts as a sinus infection that spreads to the meninges.
- *Signs and symptoms:* "The worst headache of my life," stiff neck (nuchal rigidity), lethargy, seizures, vomiting, confusion, and high fever. Infants may be febrile or irritable, may cry, may have bulging fontanels or **non-blanching rash** (**purpura**), may vomit, and may have a poor appetite.
    - **Kernig's sign** is indicative of meningitis (low back/posterior thigh pain with hip flexion and gradual knee extension).
- *Interventions:* Place the patient on droplet precautions during triage until test results return negative. Anticipate following orders: administer antipyretics; document frequent vital signs and neurologic assessments; prepare a complete blood count, blood cultures, metabolic panel, and coagulation studies; set up for lumbar puncture; and administer IV fluids and medications (mannitol, steroids, antibiotics, vasopressors, and/or inotropes).
    - Bacterial meningitis reveals a cloudy cerebrospinal fluid (CSF) with elevated white blood cell count greater than 1,000 cells/mm^3 and low glucose. It is more serious, has an acute onset, and requires antibiotics such as vancomycin, ceftriaxone sodium (Rocephin), and rifampin. Educate the patient that rifampin is an antibiotic that turns urine and tears orange.
    - Viral meningitis reveals a mildly elevated white blood cell count of 100 to 1,000 cells/mm^3 or greater and normal glucose in the CSF. It may require antiviral medication, has a gradual onset, but usually resolves on its own.

Essential Facts

Providers will tell you that positioning is key for obtaining a good lumbar puncture. For better positioning during a sitting lumbar puncture, place a step stool under the patient's feet. This brings the knees closer to the chest. To avoid complications such as infection, headache, and backache, have the patient lie flat on their back for a few hours after the procedure.

- Ensure each CSF collection tube is labeled correctly:
    - Tube 1—glucose and protein
    - Tube 2—cell count with differential
    - Tube 3—Gram stain culture
    - Tube 4—repeat cell count with differential or other studies

Notes: ____

____

____

____

____

____

____

____

____

____

____

____

____

____

____

____

____

____

____

____

____

INFLUENZA

Influenza A, B, C, and D are seasonal viruses that typically infect between the months of November and March. Cases may be mild or severe and even lead to death, especially in those who are very young, old, immunocompromised, or pregnant or have other chronic medical conditions. It is estimated that 3 to 5 million people catch the influenza annually. About 290,000 to 650,000 people die globally from respiratory illnesses related to the flu.

- *Causes:* Respiratory droplet contact with an infected person via coughing and sneezing.
- *Signs and symptoms:* Sudden high **fevers** above 100 °F, chills, body aches, weakness, headache, congestion, **cough**, sore throat, and loss of appetite. In more severe cases, the patient may have signs of pneumonia, respiratory distress, or even respiratory failure.
- *Interventions:* **Ensure that the patient in the waiting room uses a mask and initiate droplet airborne isolation precautions per hospital protocol.** In mild cases, anticipate orders to obtain a flu swab and discharge home with antiviral prescriptions. In more severe cases, chest x-rays, IV fluid hydration, nebulized respiratory treatments, blood counts, metabolic panels, arterial blood gases, bilevel positive airway pressure or intubation, and hospital admission may be ordered.
  - Discharge instructions should include resting at home, oral hydration, vitamin C, treating the symptoms, and remaining away from work or school until afebrile for at least 24 hours. **Recommend annual vaccination, covering coughs, and good handwashing to prevent the spread of flu next time.**

Notes: ____

____

____

____

____

____

____

____

HIV/AIDS

HIV is a virus that attacks the immune system, allowing other pathogens to invade the body. AIDS is a chronic, life-threatening condition caused by HIV. In the A&E, we treat acute complications of AIDS.

- *Causes:* Contamination by HIV through blood or body fluid exchange.
- *Signs and symptoms:* Early manifestations are similar to cold and flu symptoms. Later symptoms include weight loss, fever, shortness of breath, mouth ulcers, cough, sores that would not heal, and swollen lymph nodes.
  - Abnormally low CD4 lymphocyte count may be present.
  - Common opportunistic infections include bacterial pneumonia, tuberculosis, herpes, human papillomavirus, thrush, cryptococcal meningitis, *Pneumocystis carinii* pneumonia, Kaposi's sarcoma, and non-Hodgkin's lymphoma.
- *Interventions:* Anticipate orders to treat opportunistic infections, maintain appropriate isolation depending on complications, monitor vital signs, administer acetaminophen for fever, prepare a complete blood count, perform HIV testing (enzyme-linked immunosorbent assay and Western blot tests) for unknown cases, request chest x-ray, culture wounds, and obtain IV access.

Notes: ____

____

____

____

____

____

____

____

Essential Facts

- Some states require HIV testing to be offered to A&E patients as part of their HIV screening assessment tool.
- Patients taking corticosteroids will have an elevated white blood cell count.

HEPATITIS

Hepatitis is an inflammation or infection of the liver.

- *Causes:* Alcohol abuse; overdose of medications; IV drug abuse; autoimmune disorders; contaminated food or water; and presence of hepatitis A, B, C, D, or E virus.
  - *Hepatitis A:* Contracted via the fecal/oral route; children are typically asymptomatic.
  - *Hepatitis B:* Contracted via blood or body fluids.
  - *Hepatitis C:* Contracted via blood or body fluid, commonly in IV drug abusers.
  - *Hepatitis D:* Contracted via blood or body fluids and requires coinfection of hepatitis B.
  - *Hepatitis E:* Contracted via the fecal/oral route with higher mortality rate than hepatitis A.
- *Signs and symptoms:* Patients may be asymptomatic or have ascites, chills, fever, malaise, jaundice, elevated liver enzymes, right upper quadrant abdominal pain, dark urine, anorexia, diarrhea or constipation, and nausea and vomiting. The patient often looks like Big Bird—yellow all over with a big round belly.
- *Interventions:* Anticipate orders to medicate for pain, nausea, and vomiting; administer vaccine or immunoglobulin; complete a basic metabolic panel; perform a liver function test and coagulation studies; check for abnormal bleeding; and educate the patient to stop any alcohol consumption or use of acetaminophen.

Notes: ____

____

____

____

____

____

____

____

____

____

CELLULITIS/ABSCESS/METHICILLIN-RESISTANT *STAPHYLOCOCCUS AUREUS*

Abscesses are pockets of skin infection that look like giant pimples ranging in size from a marble to a golf ball or larger. Patients with diabetes are at higher risk for cellulitis and poor healing.

- *Causes:* Most abscesses are caused by methicillin-resistant *Staphylococcus aureus* (MRSA). Others may come from other types of bacteria, clogged hair follicles, or clogged pores.
- *Signs and symptoms:* Pain, redness and warmth to affected area, proximal red streaks, pus, and/or fever.
- *Interventions:* Anticipate orders to maintain **contact isolation**; prepare the patient for possible incision and drainage of abscess; if appropriate, pack the wound, bandage the wound, and administer antibiotics and warm compresses.
  - Educate the patient on how to prevent the spread of MRSA (wash hands and bleach everything). MRSA lives dormant under fingernails and in nostrils. This is why your mom said, "Don't pick your nose"! Providers may prescribe antibiotic ointment to apply inside nostrils.

Notes: ____

____

____

____

____

____

____

____

____

____

____

____

____

FEBRILE NEUTROPENIA

A patient with febrile neutropenia is immunocompromised with a fever or a possible infection.

- *Causes:* These are usually patients receiving chemotherapy. For them, a low-grade fever, say 99.9 °F, is of concern because their immune systems are too weak to handle it.
- *Signs and symptoms:* Fever and possibly cold- or flu-like symptoms.
- *Interventions:* Reverse isolation with neutropenic precautions. During triage or when the patient is in the waiting room, provide the patient with a mask for their own protection until placed in isolation room. Monitor vital signs; anticipate orders to administer acetaminophen or ibuprofen (for fever) and antibiotics, prepare a complete blood count, obtain an IV access, and prepare for possible admission.

Notes: ____

____

____

____

____

____

____

____

____

____

____

____

____

____

TICK-BORNE ILLNESSES

These are infectious diseases caused by ticks.

Lyme disease: A *Borrelia burgdorferi* bacterial infection (see Figure 13.1).

- *Causes:* Usually spread by deer ticks.
- *Signs and symptoms:* May vary by individual but commonly include a "bull's-eye" rash at the site of tick bite and flu-like symptoms (fever, chills, joint pain, fatigue, and swollen lymph nodes). Neurologic problems may be a late sign and include ascending paralysis, Bell's palsy, dizziness, nerve pain, ataxia, and extremity numbness. Bacteria may spread to the heart, resulting in myocarditis and atrioventricular block.
- *Interventions:* Remove all ticks and administer antibiotics (e.g., doxycycline or amoxicillin) as ordered. Temporary pacemaker may be needed for 1 to 6 weeks if myocarditis has occurred.

Notes: ____

____

____

____

____

____

____

____

____

____

____

____

____

____

____

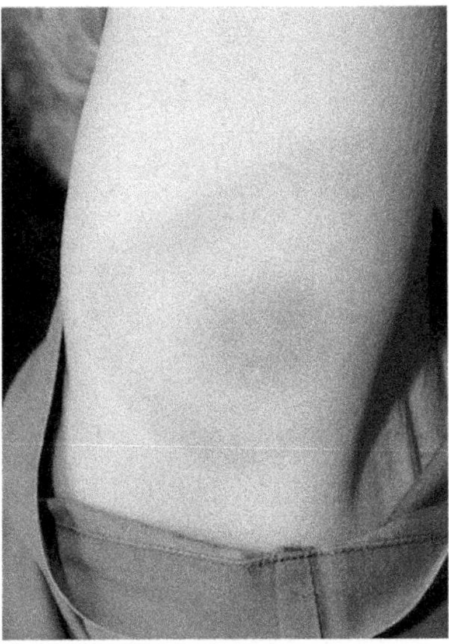

Figure 13.1 Bull's-eye rash of Lyme disease.
Source: Centers for Disease Control and Prevention.

Rocky Mountain spotted fever: A bacterial infection transmitted by ticks (see Figure 13.2).

- *Causes:* Bite from tick contaminated with *Rickettsia rickettsii* bacteria.
- *Signs and symptoms:* High fever, tick bite 2 to 14 days earlier, poor appetite, headache, body aches, nausea and vomiting, abdominal pain, fatigue, and red spotted rash in 90% of cases.
- *Interventions:* Anticipate orders to remove all ticks; obtain complete blood count, metabolic panel, liver enzymes, and coagulation studies; administer antibiotics (e.g., doxycycline) as ordered.

Notes: ____

____

____

____

____

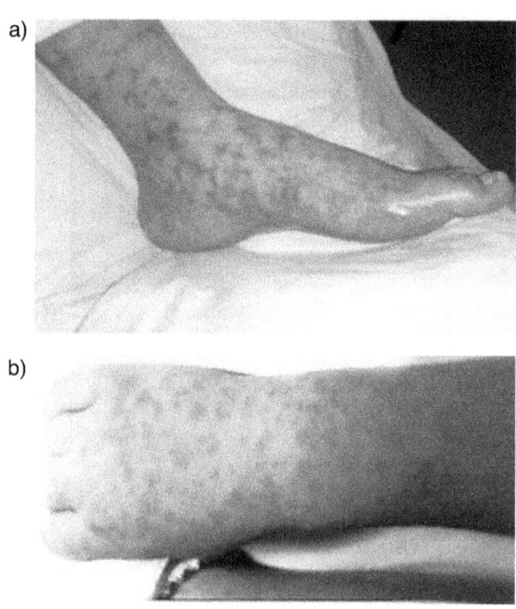

Figure 13.2 Rocky Mountain spotted fever rash of (a) foot and (b) hand.
Source: www.cdc.gov/rmsf

Notes: _________________________________

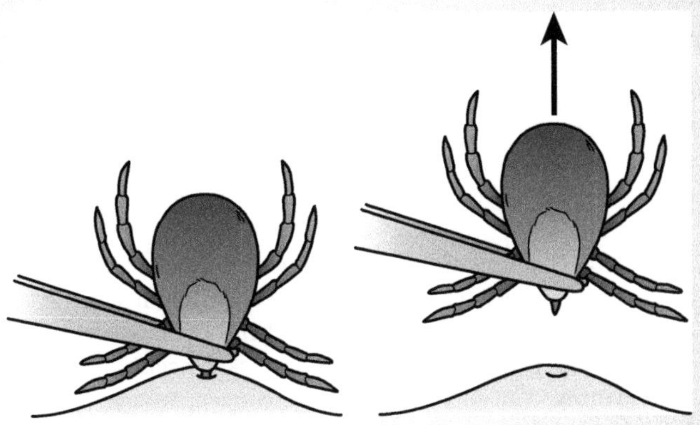

Figure 13.3 Tick removal.

- For easy tick removal, use tweezers and grasp the head portion (see Figure 13.3).
- Pull steadily and evenly from its head.
- If any mouth pieces remain, use tweezers to remove them.
- Thoroughly cleanse the tick bite area with soap and water, with antiseptic solution, or with rubbing alcohol.
- Dispose by flushing down the toilet.

Notes: ____

____

____

____

____

____

____

____

____

____

TOXIC SHOCK SYNDROME

Toxic shock syndrome is a life-threatening *S. aureus* or group A beta-hemolytic strep bacterial infection.

- *Causes:* May occur with recent surgery, burns, or open wounds and the use of tampons vaginally or nasally. The toxins released from these two bacteria can cause the patient to go into septic shock *very rapidly*—sometimes right before your eyes.
- *Signs and symptoms:* Similar to septic shock but with faster onset; includes sudden high fever; hypotension; headache; confusion; tachycardia; nausea, vomiting, and diarrhea; sunburn-like rash with desquamation (skin peeling); fatigue; and seizures.
- *Interventions:* You must work rapidly. Place the patient on contact isolation. Monitor for vital signs; anticipate orders to insert a large-bore IV access for administration of IV isotonic fluid bolus and, as soon as possible, antibiotics; place the patient in the modified Trendelenburg position for hypotension; prepare a complete blood count; take blood cultures; remove any foreign body in any body cavity and get a wound culture (if source is vaginal, prepare for pelvic exam with cultures); give norepinephrine or dopamine for hypotension and antipyretics; prepare for possible ICU admission.
  - If the patient is stable, try to obtain blood cultures before giving antibiotics. If unstable, give the antibiotics now!

Notes: ____

____

____

____

____

____

____

____

____

____

____

TUBERCULOSIS

In its *active phase,* tuberculosis is a life-threatening bacterial infection that commonly attacks the lungs but can attack other organs as well. Persons at high risk include those who live in homeless shelters, unsanitary conditions, nursing homes, or correctional institutions. IV drug users, healthcare workers, immunocompromised persons, and travelers to Asia, Africa, or Latin America are also at risk.

- *Causes: Mycobacterium tuberculosis* is spread via droplets, so negative pressure airborne isolation is necessary. In its dormant stage, tuberculosis is not contagious, and the patient is asymptomatic.
- *Signs and symptoms:* The patient can be asymptomatic or have a cough lasting several weeks; coughing up blood (hemoptysis), fever, night sweats, and fatigue are the symptoms.
- *Interventions:* **Screen patients for tuberculosis in triage** and provide a mask to patients suspected of infection. Then place the patient in a room on respiratory isolation. Anticipate orders to obtain IV access, request a chest x-ray, obtain a complete blood count, administer antibiotics (e.g., isoniazid and rifampin), and prepare for possible admission. Instruct family members and caregivers to get tuberculosis testing. Be sure to document the time the droplet-negative pressure isolation was initiated and if a mask was provided in triage or in the waiting room.

Notes: ____

____

____

____

____

____

Question: What drug besides phenazopyridine (Pyridium) makes your urine orange?
Answer: *Rifampin.*

To remember drugs used to treat tuberculosis, just remember **RIPE**—**r**ifampin, **i**soniazid, **p**yrazinamide, and **e**thambutol.

PARASITIC AND INSECT INFESTATIONS

SCABIES (*SARCOPTES SCABIEI* VAR. HOMINIS)

Scabies are little, contagious mites that burrow under the skin. Sometimes just saying the word "scabies" out loud will psychologically make you and your colleagues start to feel itchy.

- *Causes:* Despite the psychological itching, it is not possible to get scabies by simply being in the same room with the patient. They are transmitted by **prolonged skin-to-skin contact** from an infected person, their clothes, or their bed linens.
- *Signs and symptoms:* Within 2 to 6 weeks, an extremely itchy red rash with white pimple or thread-like burrows appears. This rash can occur all over, especially in skin folds of the body, such as web spaces between toes and fingers or near joints.
- *Interventions:* Anticipate orders for **contact precautions** and a prescription for topical scabicide cream such as permethrin 5% (Elimite), crotamiton lotion 10%, sulfur (5%–10%), or lindane 1% (Kwell). Discharge instructions should include applying scabicide cream to the entire body from the neck down, including all web spaces and folds to clean skin (after shower or bath) daily for the prescribed length of time. To avoid reinfection, it is important to instruct all partners or persons who had skin-to-skin contact in the past month to be examined and treated at the same time. All bed linens and clothing should be laundered in hot water or hot dryer. Non-washable items may be sealed in plastic bags for 72 hours.

Notes: ____

BEDBUGS

Cimex lectularius are tiny 1-to-7-mm flat bugs that feed on human and animal blood while they sleep. While it is not common to treat bedbug bites in the A&E, sometimes bedbugs hitch a ride on our patients and their belongings when they come to the A&E. If not identified, this can quickly become an infectious disease problem for the entire hospital.

- *Causes:* Bedbugs can be picked up easily when traveling, from hotels, buses, trains, luggage, cruise ships, and dorm rooms. They can hide in the seams of fabric mattresses, box springs, head-boards, dressers, seats, wall paper, and clothes in suitcases.

- *Signs and symptoms:* **Painless** itchy bugbites to face, neck, arms, legs, or other body parts while sleeping. Bedbugs or their exoskeletons may be found in the folds and seams of the mattress and sheets.
- *Interventions:* Initiate contact precautions and contact your hospital infection preventionist. Topical creams may be prescribed to the patient to help with itching and healing. Antibiotics may be ordered if secondary infection occurs. If the patient is to be admitted, special environmental interventions may be implemented, such as sealing all the patient's belongings into plastic bags while having the patient shower. The patient's belongings may be taken home or placed in the patient's car. Decontamination of the room with insecticides may be implemented after the patient leaves the room.

Notes: ____

MYIASIS: MAGGOT WOUND INFESTATION

While certain species of fly larvae are helpful because the eat only necrotic, or dead, tissues, other species are indiscriminate and will eat both healthy and dead tissue. It is not very common, but I have seen it a few times in the A&E, more commonly in nursing home patients or homeless patients.

- *Causes:* Occurs when a fly lays its eggs in an open flesh wound or on a mosquito that then bites a human or when the larvae themselves burrow directly into the skin.
- *Signs and symptoms:* A closed or open wound with maggots inside.
- *Interventions:* Maintain standard/universal precautions. Prepare for operating room admission as the maggots will need to be surgically removed and the wound debrided. Until then, anticipate orders to soak the wound in hydrogen peroxide, clean and dress the wound, and administer antibiotics and tetanus vaccine. The peroxide will kill most of the maggots prior to surgery. Consider sealing the edges of the dressing to keep the rest of the larvae contained during transfer to the operating room.

Notes: ____

FOOD AND DRINKS AT WORKSTATIONS

It is important to stay hydrated as an A&E nurse. However, the A&E environment is not the safest place for your food or drinks, not if you are trying to avoid getting sick, that is. Potential contamination may occur if food and drinks are left at workstations; therefore, **do not eat or drink in these areas**. A simple solution may be a designated hydration station. These designated areas have been determined to represent less risk for contaminated food and drinks.

Notes: ____

____

____

____

____

____

ENVIRONMENT OF CARE

Even if the bed was wiped down and new sheets were applied, many germs may linger on the call button, side rails, cabinet handles, thermometer, monitors, bedside table, otoscope handles, or light switches. It's important to make a habit of wiping down high-touch surfaces when you clean a room. Honestly, any equipment that goes from patient to patient or room to room also needs to be disinfected between patients/rooms. This includes things like blood pressure machines/cuffs, blood glucometers, and wheelchairs. Wipe the equipment thoroughly with the appropriate disinfectant; let it dry completely. Make an effort to wipe your work areas as well as the patient rooms, especially the high-touch surfaces.

Notes: ____

____

____

____

____

____

____

SUMMARY

Most A&Es do not allow new graduate nurses to triage until proper training and experience are achieved. This is partly because the triage nurses are the front line when it comes to exposure to infectious diseases. Therefore, it is crucial to thoroughly screen all patients who come through triage for infectious diseases. If an infectious disease is suspected, proper isolation must be implemented. Make sure you become familiar with your facility's isolation protocols and equipment and know how to use it. This information may seem a bit scary at first, but look around you. There are A&E nurses who have been doing this for decades! As an A&E nurse, remember that you are the first line of defense in preventing the spread of transmissible infectious disease. The key is **good handwashing**, universal precautions, triage travel screening, proper isolation, and notification of appropriate personnel.

14

Mental Health Emergencies

Mental health emergencies may not be everyone's favorite topic. We can all empathize; everyone experiences anxiety, stress, anger, and depression in their lives, but some people become suicidal, violent, or psychotic. Mental health patients may be difficult to treat at times, particularly when they engage in disruptive behavior. At times, security, antianxiety medication, seclusion, and restraints may be necessary for short periods of time to maintain patient safety. However, restraints should be a last resort after the least restrictive measures have been attempted. Restraint legal documentation requirements can be intense and vary according to the purpose (medical/nonviolent vs. violent behavior). Take the time to learn the various restraint documentation requirements during orientation. Be aware that state suicide intent documentation does not always necessitate restraints and vice versa. **Your priority must always be to maintain safety for yourself, your staff members, your patient, and other patients.** However, you will find that most mental health patients respond better if you listen, respect their personal space, and educate them on all procedures clearly and early on.

During this part of your orientation, locate and become familiar with:

- Your state's and facility's seclusion and restraint policies
- Restraint and seclusion forms
- Legal suicidal intent documents
- Transfer policies to mental health facilities
- Local mental health counselors and facilities

- Your facility's security and its codes
- Nonviolent crisis intervention training
- Medications to know: lorazepam (Ativan), haloperidol (Haldol), and ziprasidone (Geodon)

ANXIETY

Anxiety is a vague feeling of apprehension, tension, and uneasiness that can be divided into four levels: mild, moderate, severe, and panic.

- *Causes:* Usually some sort of stressor, but it varies with the individual and their circumstances.
- *Signs and symptoms by level:*
  - *Mild:* Minimal muscle tension; normal vital signs; constricted normal pupils; random controlled thoughts; and appearance of calm.
  - *Moderate:* Normal to slightly elevated vital signs; tension; excited behavior; alertness; optimum state for problem-solving and learning; attentiveness; and energization.
  - *Severe:* Flight-or-fight response; tachycardia; tachypnea; hypertension; diaphoretic; urinary urgency; diarrhea; dry mouth; dilated pupils; difficulty in problem-solving; feeling overwhelmed; and decreased appetite.
  - *Panic:* Faint feeling or syncope from sympathetic nervous system release; pallor; hyperventilation; hypertension; pain; weakness; lack of coordination; choking or gasping sensation; chest pressure or lump in throat; helplessness; and shortness of breath; may become angry/combative/withdrawn, tearful.
- *Interventions:* Maintain calm and private environment; reduce stimulation; stay with the patient or have a support person stay; use simple repetitive communication; encourage verbalization of feelings; administer antianxiety/analgesic medications; evaluate effectiveness of medications; and teach relaxation/breathing techniques.

Notes: ____

____

____

____

POSTTRAUMATIC STRESS DISORDER

The disorder is a reaction to overwhelmingly traumatic events.

- *Causes:* A traumatic or overwhelming event such as military combat, rape, and natural or man-made disaster.
- *Signs and symptoms:* Signs of anxiety, hyperarousal, or stress; recurring dreams or flashbacks, which may be accompanied by dissociative reactions; explosive anger; increased substance abuse; sleep disturbances; difficulty concentrating; avoidance of activities surrounding the event; and feelings of guilt.
- *Interventions:* Assess suicidal/homicidal ideations; assess anxiety levels; provide therapeutic listening; avoid judgment; and provide referrals for group or individual counseling.

Notes: ____

____

____

____

____

____

____

____

____

____

____

____

____

____

____

DEPRESSION

Depression is a state of sadness or hopelessness that affects one mentally and physically. Short periods of depression following a specific event, such as divorce or death, are natural and resolve in time. However, clinical depression related to chemical or hormonal imbalances may require medication and therapy for a period of time or a lifetime.

- *Causes:* Vary by individual and circumstances. May be the natural result of a specific event, such as divorce or death, or may be more situational. If, however, it is the result of hormonal or chemical imbalances, the condition may require prolonged treatment.
- *Signs and symptoms:* Sad mood; lack of interest in or pleasure from activities; insomnia or hypersomnia; fatigue; feelings of guilt or worthlessness; inability to think or concentrate; inability to make decisions; anorexia; and suicidal ideation or attempt.
- *Interventions:* Assess suicide risk; discuss patient's emotional state; show interest and concern; and provide choices. Antidepressants are rarely administered in the A&E; they are not usually effective for the first week or two.

Notes: ____

____

____

____

____

____

Essential Facts

- Monoamine oxidase inhibitors + alcohol = hypertensive crisis
- Monoamine oxidase inhibitors + foods that ferment (yogurt, cheeses, sour cream) = hypertensive crisis

Question: Why don't we typically discharge patients with antidepressant prescriptions?

Answer: *These patients need psychiatric follow-up and probably will not go if they are able to receive medications in the A&E.*

SUICIDE

Suicide is an intentional self-inflicted death. Suicidal actions include suicidal thoughts, threats, gestures, and/or attempts.

- *Causes:* Vary by individual and circumstance. There are, however, common risk factors: male; age older than 65 years; Caucasian; substance/physical/sexual/mental/emotional abuse; depression; family history of or prior suicide attempt; terminal or chronic illness; psychosis; living alone; recent change/loss in life; and low self-esteem.
- *Signs and symptoms:* Previous suicide attempts; verbal statements of suicidal thoughts; giving away favorite items; writing a will; depressed mood; isolated; and withdrawn.
- *Interventions:* Create a safe room for the patient; have security scan the patient with a metal detection device and remove any potentially dangerous objects or contraband from the patient and the room. Dress the patient in a suicidal safe gown and secure any personal belongings. Document according to hospital policy for high risk or suicidal patients. Engage in one-to-one observations; encourage verbal expression of feelings/thoughts; promote hope; obtain labs as ordered for medical clearance; and obtain mental health evaluation. Assessment questions are listed as follows.
  - Are you having thoughts about ending your life?
  - If you had a way, would you try to take your own life?
  - Have you ever had specific thoughts or plans about ending your own life?
  - Have you set a time or place?
  - What are these plans?
  - Do you have access to _________________________ [this method]?
  - Have you done anything or made preparations to take your own life?

Notes: ____

____

____

____

____

____

____

Sad Persons Scale

Risk Factors	Points
S—Sex	1 point if male; 0 if female
A—Age	1 point for age <20 or >44
D—Depression	1 point if present
P—Previous attempt	1 point if present
E—Ethanol abuse	1 point if present
R—Rational thinking loss	1 point if present
S—Social support lacking	1 point if present
O—Organized plan	1 point if plan is made and lethal
N—No spouse	1 if divorced, widowed, separated, or single
S—Sickness	1 if chronic, debilitating, and severe

Total Points	Risk Assessment
0–5	Low: may be safe for discharge
5–8	Moderate: possible mental health consult required
8–10	High: possible mental health admission

Essential Facts

The 20-year-old suicidal male patient who describes to you in detail how he is going to commit suicide is the most dangerous.

VIOLENT OR AGGRESSIVE BEHAVIOR

This is behavior that has harmed or may result in harm to the patient or others.

- *Causes:* Many factors can trigger aggressive behavior, including alcohol, drugs, or long waiting times in the A&E.
- *Signs and symptoms:* Loud/threatening speech; yelling profanities; bragging about past violence; demanding personality; pacing; acting tense; clenching fists; slamming/pushing/throwing objects; alcohol odor; or other unusual behavior.
- *Interventions:* It is tough, but you have to **stay calm**; speak softly/slowly/clearly; respect patient's personal space; provide brief and honest facts; be an empathetic listener; encourage patient to verbalize feelings; provide "show of force" with security if needed; restrain as last resort; medicate as ordered and as necessary; and document all interventions and behaviors.
  - There are some people you cannot make happy no matter what you do. When you have tried everything listed previously, tell the person you will find someone to help and calmly *walk away!* Then chart the person's behavior and your interventions. Notify your charge nurse or supervisor that you require assistance.

Notes: ____

____

____

____

____

____

____

____

____

____

____

PSYCHOSIS

Psychosis is defined as a grossly impaired sense of reality. It is commonly associated with schizophrenia, which usually includes "negative symptoms," such as difficulty forming social and coherent conversations.

- *Causes:* Origin may be unknown, but the patient must be medically cleared. Some brain injuries, chemical imbalances, loss, separation, rejection, and use of illicit drugs can also cause psychosis.
- *Signs and symptoms:* Delusions; hallucinations; disorganized speech or behavior; catatonia; paranoia; poverty of speech; and flat affect.
- *Interventions:* Reorient to reality; maintain calm professional manner; explain unseen noises/voices/activities clearly and simply; give haloperidol (Haldol) as ordered; and respect patient's personal space.

Notes: ____

____

____

____

____

____

____

____

____

Essential Facts

- Do not touch a patient who is hallucinating.
- The drug of choice for acute psychotic behavior is haloperidol (Haldol), administered by injection or intravenously.
- Large doses of haloperidol (Haldol) may prolong the Q-T interval; cardiac monitoring may be required.

MANIC BEHAVIOR

Manic behavior is an elevated, unstable, or irritable mood. Bipolar disorder includes manic and depressive behaviors.

- *Causes:* Bipolar disorder and drug use are common.
- *Signs and symptoms:* Euphoria; grandiosity; insomnia; flight of ideas; aggression; easily distracted; impulsive; increased motor activity; and pressured speech (i.e., very talkative). You cannot get one word in with these patients.
- *Interventions:* Reduce stimuli; obtain urine drug screen and lithium level as ordered; reorient to reality; use "show of force" as needed with security personnel for aggressive behavior; set limits on manipulative/negative behavior; and restrain as needed for safety according to policy.

Notes: ____

____

____

____

____

____

____

____

____

____

____

Essential Facts

A manic patient is at risk for harming themself or others because of reckless behavior.

SUMMARY

You should now have a better understanding of mental health emergencies and how to handle them. From sad and suicidal patients to loud and schizophrenic patients wearing lampshades on their heads, you never know what kind of mental health challenge you will face next in the A&E. Nevertheless, your mental health patients will respond better when you remain calm, speak concisely, respect personal space, and inform patients of upcoming procedures. *There are important legal issues and patient rights regarding mental health emergencies.* **Document carefully** and become familiar with your state's and facility's legal forms and policies regarding suicide, restraints, and seclusion. In addition, know how to get a hold of security personnel if you need them right away. You may find that mental health emergencies can be tough, sad, and rewarding.

15

Musculoskeletal and Wound Care Emergencies

You will definitely see all kinds of musculoskeletal and wound emergencies in the A&E. You need to be familiar with many different pieces of orthopedic equipment. In addition to using the equipment, the A&E nurse is also responsible for teaching the patient how to use the orthopedic equipment. For casts of Ortho-Glass®–type splinting, I recommend training from the manufacturer's representative. **Most manufacturers will send someone to your facility to demonstrate their products and allow employees to practice applying the splints.** Most A&E technicians are qualified to apply splints for you, but the nurse must ensure the work was done properly. **Assess and document circulation, motion, and sensation before and after splinting**. This chapter provides a brief overview of the different orthopedic and wound care emergency situations you may come across in the A&E, and how to handle them.

During this part of your orientation, locate and become familiar with:

- Ace wraps, splinting, and casting materials
- Pain scales and documentation
- Crutches
- Hare traction splints and Buck's traction
- Tube gauze and hemostatic gauze
- Finger traps and weights

- Suture supplies and dressing supplies
- Moderate/conscious sedation policy and procedure
- Tetanus vaccination policy and procedure
- Medications to know: Lidocaine 1% or 2% (with or without epinephrine), bupivacaine (Marcaine) with or without epinephrine, morphine, hydrocodone (Lortab), oxycodone (Percocet), and acetaminophen (Tylenol) with codeine

STRAINS

A strain is a pull or tear to a tendon or muscle.

- *Causes:* Injury resulting in a pull or tear to a tendon.
- *Signs and symptoms:* Pain; swelling; ecchymosis; edema; point tenderness; spasm; and decreased range of motion.
- *Interventions:* Mnemonic **PRICE** (Protect [splint, cast, sling], Rest, Ice, Compression [ace wrap], Elevate); x-ray; instruct patient on use of crutches for light to no weight bearing; and arrange orthopedic follow-up.

Notes: ____

____

____

____

____

____

____

____

____

____

____

____

SPRAINS

A sprain is a pull or tear to a ligament, commonly in the knees, ankles, and shoulders.

- *Causes:* Injury resulting in a pull or tear to a ligament.
- *Signs and symptoms:* Pain; swelling; ecchymosis; edema; point tenderness; spasm; and decreased range of motion.
- *Interventions:* Mnemonic PRICE; x-ray; instruct patient on light to no weight bearing (crutches); and arrange orthopedic follow-up.

Notes: ____

FRACTURES

A fracture is a broken bone or disruption in normal continuity of bone, cartilage, or both.

- *Types:*
  - *Closed*: Skin intact.
  - *Open*: Broken bone with break in the skin surrounding the fracture. Patient is at high risk for developing an infection in the bone (osteomyelitis).
  - *Avulsion*: Insertion site bone fragment breaks away due to forceful muscle contraction.
  - *Comminuted*: Two or more bone fragments.
  - *Depressed*: Flat bone injury due to blunt trauma.
  - *Greenstick*: Incomplete compression force-type fracture (common in school-age children).
  - *Spiral*: Twisting injury.
  - *Oblique*: Linear oblique fracture.
  - *Transverse*: Horizontal linear fracture.
  - *Segmented*: Broken in two or more places.
  - *Salter–Harris*: Fracture involving the growth plate.
  - *Boxer fracture*: Occurs to the fourth or fifth metacarpals after punching-type injury.
- *Causes:* Injury or disease process resulting in a break to the bone. Consider corresponding injuries to surrounding tissue, nerves, blood vessels, or internal organs.
- *Signs and symptoms:* Pain; tenderness; swelling; redness; ecchymosis; deformity; shortening/rotation in hip fracture; decreased range of motion; inability to bear weight; muscle spasm; crepitus; weak or absent pulses; pallor; and shock.
- *Interventions:* Administer pain medication promptly as ordered and document effectiveness; immobilize; assist in applying traction for femur fracture; remove any rings or jewelry to the fractured extremity; cover open fractures with sterile saline-soaked dressing; mnemonic PRICE; x-ray; instruct patient on light to no weight bearing (crutches); prepare for possible closed reduction; give nothing by mouth; give instructions for possible surgical repair; teach cast care instructions and crutch training; check peripheral pulses; anticipate orders to start intravenous (IV) access; possibly give IV fluids and tetanus immunization if open fracture; and arrange orthopedic follow-up.

Notes: ____

Essential Facts

If a patient with a long bone fracture suddenly develops an altered mental status, visual disturbances, respiratory distress, tachycardia, petechial chest rash, or thrombocytopenia, consider fat embolism syndrome.

Question: Pneumothorax or great vessel injury may occur with which type of fracture?
Answer: *Clavicle (collar bone) fracture.*

Question: How long does it take a bone to heal?
Answer: *About 6 weeks.*

Question: What other x-ray should be ordered for the patient who has bilateral heel fractures after falling 13 ft off a ladder and landing on their feet?
Answer: *Check the L-spine.*

Question: Which bones, if broken, can lead to hemorrhagic shock?
Answer: *Pelvis and femur.*

Question: How much blood can be lost in one femur fracture?
Answer: *Up to 1,500 mL.*

Question: When applying a thumb spica Ortho-Glass splint, how should you position the hand?
Answer: *As if the patient were holding a cup or soda can.*

DISLOCATIONS AND SUBLUXATIONS

Dislocations and subluxations occur when a joint is pulled out of place.

- *Causes:* Injury or movement resulting in joint dislocation.
- *Signs and symptoms:* Severe joint pain; joint deformity/asymmetry; decreased or absent range of motion; weak or absent pulse; edema; and shortening of extremity.
- *Interventions:* Anticipate orders to obtain x-ray films, prepare for conscious/moderate sedation for closed reduction, apply ice pack, start IV access, prepare a neurovascular assessment, immobilize joint postreduction, and obtain postreduction x-ray.

Notes: ____

____

____

____

____

____

____

____

____

____

____

____

____

____

____

____

____

____

____

AMPUTATION

Amputation is a partial or complete separation of a limb.

- *Causes:* Injury/trauma resulting in separation of a limb.
- *Signs and symptoms:* Completely or partially detached extremity.
- *Interventions:* Treat airway, breathing, and circulation (ABCs) first. Administer oxygen and initiate two large-bore IV accesses. Wrap amputated part in sterile saline-soaked gauze and place in sterile plastic bag or container. Place bag or container on crushed ice and water. **Never put amputated part directly on ice.** Control bleeding; apply sterile saline-soaked dressing to amputation site; anticipate orders to administer pain meds/ antibiotics/tetanus immunization and evaluate effectiveness of medications; and prepare for surgery.

Notes: ____

____

____

____

____

____

____

____

____

____

____

Essential Facts

Do not forget to properly label the amputated part.

COMPARTMENT SYNDROME

This occurs when a compartment of the limb becomes full of fluid or blood, thereby hindering circulation to that extremity.

- *Causes:* Usually occurs with trauma.
- *Signs and symptoms:* The six **P**s: **P**ain, **P**ressure, **P**aresthesia, **P**ulselessness, **P**aralysis, and **P**allor.
- *Interventions:* Administer antiinflammatory drugs as ordered; **elevate the affected limb to the level of the heart;** and reassess neurovascular status. Prepare for intramuscular pressure measurements (normal is 0–8 mmHg) and possible emergency fasciotomy. Ice is contraindicated as it will compromise circulation. Discharge teaching should include instructions to return for any increasing pain, pallor, or decreased circulation below the cast or splint.

Notes: ____

____

____

____

____

____

____

____

____

____

____

____

Question: What would happen if you elevated a limb with compartment syndrome above the level of the heart?

Answer: *Blood flow and profusion would decrease compromising circulation to the extremity.*

LACERATIONS VERSUS CUTS

Lacerations are breaks or tears in the skin due to blunt trauma. Cuts occur from sharp objects.

- *Causes:* Everything from pieces of glass, knives, and razors to umbrellas, coffee tables, and baseball bats. You name it; almost anything can cause a laceration or cut.
- *Signs and symptoms:* Bleeding, cut, and open wound. An arterial laceration will intermittently squirt blood with each pulse. If a vein is cut, it will constantly ooze. Superficial lacerations are easily repaired in the A&E. Deep wounds through the muscle fascia or tendons may require a plastic surgeon.
- *Interventions:* Apply pressure to control bleeding; update tetanus shot if greater than 5 years since last one; cleanse wound with chlorhexidine soap; prepare patient for wound closure with Dermabond, Steri-strips, or sutures per provider order; bandage accordingly.

Notes: ____

____

____

____

____

____

____

____

Question: When setting up for suture repair of the ear, nose, penis, fingers, or toes, should you use lidocaine with epinephrine?
Answer: *No.*

Question: What supplies are needed for suture setup?
Answer: *Suture tray, sutures, povidone-iodine (Betadine)/ChloraPrep, saline, lidocaine, Chux, and sterile gloves.*

Question: What are three shots that can be given in the deltoid?
Answer: *Tetanus/diphtheria, rabies vaccine, and the flu shot.*

BURNS

A burn is a breakdown in the skin.

- *Causes:* Chemicals; sun; heat; radiation; fire; electrical; or even cold substances such as dry ice.
- *Signs and symptoms:*
  - *First degree:* Superficial pink color or redness; pain; blanches; and warmth to area.
  - *Second degree:* Partial thickness, redness; blistering; break in first layer of skin down to second layer of skin; and pain.
  - *Third degree:* White waxy areas or charred black areas to skin; painless; full thickness: all layers of skin affected; requires skin grafts.
  - *Fourth degree:* Painless, full-thickness burn extending down into muscle layers and bone requiring amputation.
- *Interventions:* Stop burning process with tap water. Check ABCs first. Patient may have smoke/burn inhalation or carbon monoxide poisoning; consider proactive intubation. For minor burns, give pain medication as ordered; cleanse burns with chlorhexidine soap and saline; and apply antibiotic ointment or silver sulfadiazine (Silvadene) cream and nonadherent dressings. Screen the patient for possible abuse. If it is a **major burn**, do not apply creams or ointments; instead, **cover with dry sterile drape or clean sheet**, start IV access, give analgesics, and prepare for admission to burn center. Use the rule of nines, rule of palm, or modified Lund and Browder chart to determine total burn surface area (TBSA).

Notes: ____

____

____

____

____

____

____

____

____

____

Question: Why are wet-to-dry dressings contraindicated in patients with major burns?
Answer: *Wet-to-dry dressings may cause hypothermia.*

Question: When estimating a burn with the rule of palm, should you use the patient's hand or your hand to measure? What percentage is one hand?
Answer: *Use the patient's hand, including fingers. The size of the patient's wrist to fingertips measures about 1% of the burned area.*

Question: If a 100-kg patient sustains 50% TBSA, what rate should you begin their IV lactated Ringer's fluid bolus? For burns >20%, TBSA uses the following formula: kg × 2 mL × %TBSA = IV fluids over 24 hours; give half over first 8 hours.
Answer: *100 × 2 × 50 = 10,000 mL over 24 hr; 10,000/2 = 5,000 mL; 5,000 mL/8 hr = 625 mL/hr for first 8 hours.*

Figure 15.1 shows the "rule of nines" for adult burn victims. This is a fast way to determine a patient's percentage of burned surfaces using multiples of nine.

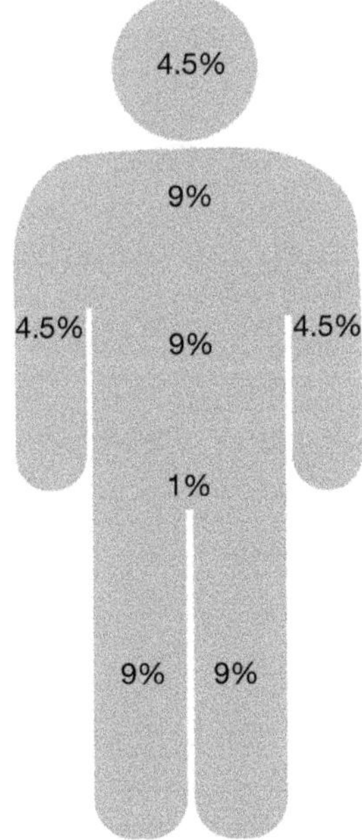

Figure 15.1 Rule of nines.

OSTEOMYELITIS

An infection of the bone.

- *Causes:* Direct contamination from open fractures, penetrating wounds, or surgical procedures. The longer the surgery, the greater the risk. *Staphylococcus aureus* is a common source.
- *Signs and symptoms:* Fever, pain, or tenderness over infected area; edema; redness; drainage; and elevated white blood cell count (WBC).
- *Interventions:* Anticipate orders to immobilize the extremity, obtain blood and wound cultures, administer IV antibiotics, perform bone scan, assist with surgical debridement, and monitor for development of sepsis.

Notes: ____

____

____

____

____

____

____

____

____

____

____

____

____

____

____

____

____

____

RHABDOMYOLYSIS

Rhabdomyolysis is a complex medical condition that results from a significant cellular damage or lysis to muscle tissues. Excessive amounts of **myoglobin**, creatinine kinase, electrolytes, and lactate dehydrogenase are released into the blood stream and extracellular tissues. Because myoglobin is a large molecule, it gets trapped in the renal tubules resulting in **renal failure**.

- *Causes:* Most commonly musculoskeletal crush injury trauma. However, infection, toxins, electrolyte imbalances, prolonged immobilization, extreme exercise, third-degree burns, snake venom, metabolic disorders, muscle ischemia, and hyperthermia can also lead to rhabdomyolysis.
- *Signs and symptoms:* Classic triad
  1. **Tea colored (red or brownish) urine** (due to **myoglobinuria**)
  2. Muscular pain (soft-tissue damage and bruising)
  3. Muscular weakness or paralysis
- *Interventions:* Anticipate orders for aggressive IV fluid resuscitation, large-bore IV access, urinalysis, creatinine kinase levels, hemoglobin levels, and metabolic panel; monitor and document urine output, use cardiac monitoring, provide pharmacologic and nonpharmacologic pain relief, and prepare for admission and, in severe cases, dialysis.

Notes: ____

____

____

____

____

____

____

____

____

____

____

SUMMARY

You now have a better understanding of musculoskeletal and wound care emergencies, their symptoms, and treatments. Be sure to familiarize yourself with the musculoskeletal and wound care supplies at your local facility. Thoroughly document your assessments, being sure to include distal pulses, capillary refills, deformities, symmetry, whether bleeding is controlled, and when and how the injury occurred. Use personal protective equipment, especially with arterial bleeds. Arterial bleeds have been known to squirt across the room. In case this happens, and your clothes get soiled, it is also a good idea to **keep an extra pair of scrubs in your locker**. Teach patients the importance of an orthopedic follow-up; the A&E visit goal is to stabilize, and small fractures may not be visible until swelling subsides.

16

Neurologic Emergencies

The neurologic system is a critical piece of the human puzzle. It is fascinating and fragile. There are many different forms of neurologic emergencies. In the A&E, you may see anything from **head trauma with grand mal seizures to Bell's palsy.** It is important to get a good history and neurologic assessment on these patients. This chapter helps you learn the major neurologic emergencies and how to handle them.

During this part of your orientation, locate and become familiar with:

- Acute stroke protocol for your facility
- How to become National Institutes of Health Stroke Scale (NIHSS) certified online
- Neurologic assessment tools (NIHSS and Glasgow Coma Scale)
- Alteplase (tPA) administration guidelines
- Medications to know: heparin, warfarin (Coumadin), nitroglycerin, sodium nitroprusside (Nipride), phenytoin (Dilantin), diazepam (Valium), and lorazepam (Ativan)

PLAN FOR THE WORST, HOPE FOR THE BEST

I will never forget a patient who took me by surprise. He came in unconscious and postictal from a witnessed seizure with no history available and no family. We were treating him for a routine seizure when he suddenly became hypertensive with multiple seizures, and we learned of his history of uncontrolled hypertension. He was having a massive hemorrhagic stroke—and not just a routine seizure! He needed a head CT scan super-stat!

ACUTE STROKE (CEREBROVASCULAR ACCIDENT)

A stroke is an interruption of cerebral circulation, also known as a "cerebrovascular accident." An acute stroke is marked by an onset of neurologic symptoms within the past 48 hours and is considered a time-sensitive emergency. Time = brain tissue. The three classifications of strokes are listed in the following, along with their causes, manifestations, and interventions.

Ischemic Stroke

- *Causes:* Clot; thrombus; embolus; compression; or spasm. Large artery atherosclerosis, chronic hypertension, high cholesterol, obesity, atrial fibrillation, and diabetes contribute to ischemic strokes.
- *Signs and symptoms:* Usually occur while sleeping. Symptoms, which vary depending on location, magnitude, and duration, include arm drift; pupil changes; paralysis; facial droop; weakness; nausea and vomiting; hearing loss; headache; altered mental status; aphasia; dysphasia; receptive aphasia; visual disturbances; vertigo; ataxia; symptoms of increased intracranial pressure; and seizure.
- *Interventions:* Follow hospital stroke protocol (usually **4.5-hour tPA [alteplase] window** or **24-hour thrombectomy** window from onset of symptoms to treatment); maintain patent airway; monitor cardiac rhythm and blood pressure (BP); insert two large-bore intravenous (IV) accesses; administer oxygen; activate stroke team; and obtain emergent CT scan of the head. Give antihypertensive medications as ordered if systolic BP (SBP) is >185 mmHg and diastolic BP (DBP) is >110 mmHg. Perform coagulation studies and EKG, but these should not delay tPA

administration. Obtain accurate weight, blood glucose, and frequent neurologic assessments per hospital protocol. For patients who are not alteplase candidates, give anticoagulants (e.g., heparin, warfarin [Coumadin]). If patient meets criteria, give antithrombotics (alteplase, urokinase, and streptokinase) as ordered. Prepare for admission to an intensive care or stroke unit for monitoring.

Notes: ____

Giving Alteplase

1. Establish two large-bore IV accesses.
2. Complete inclusion/exclusion criteria checklist.
3. Calculate the total dose with second nurse, doctor, or pharmacist: 0.9 mg/kg (maximum dose 90 mg).
4. Separate 10% of the total dose to give as an IV bolus over 1 minute.
5. Give remaining 90% as a continuous infusion over 60 minutes.
6. Give alteplase as early as possible. Better outcomes can be expected if given within 1.5 hours.
7. If the patient develops severe headache, acute hypertension, nausea, or vomiting or has a worsening neurologic examination, discontinue the infusion and obtain emergency head CT scan.
8. Measure BP and perform neurologic assessments every 15 minutes during and after IV alteplase infusion for 2 hours, then every 30 minutes for 6 hours, then hourly until 24 hours after IV alteplase treatment.
9. Increase the frequency of BP measurements if SBP is >180 mmHg or if DBP is >105 mmHg; administer antihypertensive medications to maintain BP at or below these levels.
10. Delay placement of nasogastric tubes, indwelling bladder catheters, or intra-arterial pressure catheters if the patient can be safely managed without them.
11. Obtain a follow-up CT or MRI scan at 24 hours after IV alteplase before starting anticoagulants or antiplatelet agents.

Notes: ____

____

____

____

Alteplase Inclusion/Exclusion Criteria

° YES	Diagnosed with ischemic stroke causing measurable and disabling neurologic deficit
° YES	Onset of symptoms ≤3–4.5 hrs
° NO	Age ≥18 years of age
° NO	Head trauma/stroke in past 3 months
° NO	Subarachnoid hemorrhage symptoms
° NO	Intracranial hemorrhage history
° NO	Intracranial neoplasm/AV malformation/aneurysm/multilobar infarction
° NO	Recent intracranial/intraspinal surgery
° NO	Elevated BP ≥185/110
° NO	Active or acute internal bleeding
° NO	Takes anticoagulants with INR >1.7 or PT <15
° NO	Blood glucose <50

Note: Provider may consider other relative exclusion criteria not listed in table. AV, arteriovenous; BP, blood pressure; INR, international normalized ratio; PT, prothrombin time.

Alteplase Door to Needle Goal ≤ 30 Minutes

Table 16.1

American Heart Association: Target Stroke Goals	
≤2.5 minutes	*Establish symptom onset time, support ABCs, **A&E provider at bedside***
≤5 minutes	***Stroke team arrival***
<10 minutes	*Obtain accurate weight, IV access, and blood glucose; order head CT; complete neurologic/stroke assessment and transfer to radiology*
≤15 minutes	***CT initiated,** assess tPA exclusion criteria*
≤25 minutes	***CT result obtained,** review risks and benefits of fibrinolytic therapy, order tPA bolus, and infusion*
<30 minutes	*tPA bolus, and infusion given to eligible patients*

ABCs, airway, breathing, and circulation; IV, intravenous; tPA, alteplase.

Notes: ____

Hemorrhagic Stroke

- *Causes:* Rupture of cerebral blood vessel. Chronic hypertension, arteriovenous (AV) malformations, tumors, bleeding abnormalities, and aneurysm ruptures also contribute to hemorrhagic strokes.

- *Signs and symptoms:* Often occur suddenly upon waking or shortly thereafter. Symptoms, which vary depending on location, magnitude, and duration, include arm drift; pupil changes; paralysis; facial droop; weakness; nausea and vomiting; hearing loss; headache; altered mental status; aphasia; dysphasia; receptive aphasia; visual disturbances; vertigo; ataxia; symptoms of increased intracranial pressure; and seizure.
- *Interventions:* Follow hospital stroke protocol; maintain patent airway; monitor cardiac rhythm and BP; administer oxygen; anticipate orders for CT scan of the head; give antihypertensive medications to maintain SBP to 150; and perform coagulation studies, glucose, EKG, and frequent neurologic assessments. Consider surgical intervention. Prepare for operating room admission with neurosurgeon or transfer as ordered.

Notes: ____

Transient Ischemic Attack

A mini stroke, also known as a "transient ischemic attack," is a temporary interruption of cerebral blood flow that resolves on its own.

- *Causes:* Temporary interruption of blood supply from a clot, spasm, or cerebral bleeding.
- *Signs and symptoms:* Symptoms, which vary depending on location, magnitude, and duration, persist less than 24 hours without permanent neurologic deficit. They include arm drift; pupil changes; paralysis; facial droop; weakness; nausea and vomiting; hearing loss; headache; altered mental status; aphasia; dysphasia; receptive aphasia; visual disturbances; vertigo; ataxia; symptoms of increased intracranial pressure; and seizure.
- *Interventions:* Follow hospital stroke protocol (usually a 4.5-hour window from onset of symptoms to treatment; see Table 16.1); maintain patent airway; watch cardiac and BP monitor; administer oxygen; anticipate orders for CT scan of the head, antihypertensive medications if SBP is >185 mmHg and DBP is >110 mmHg (do not lower BP too fast!), coagulation studies, EKG, and frequent neurologic assessments; and prepare for admission. If patient arrived more than 4.5 hours but less than 24 hours from symptom onset, they may be eligible for emergent thrombectomy.

Notes: ______________________________

____

____

____

____

____

Question: What is alteplase (tPA)?
Answer: *It is a protein that helps convert plasminogen to plasmin, a major enzyme responsible for clot breakdown. It is approved for ischemic strokes. An accurate weight must be obtained.*

Essential Facts

To triage a stroke, quickly just remember the **BEFAST** assessment (**B**alance, **E**yes, **F**ace, **A**rm, **S**peech, and **T**ime).

During triage of a stroke patient, it is vital to assess the last known well time. This will help you determine if the stroke is acute.

Question: What do you give for warfarin (Coumadin) overdose?
Answer: *Vitamin K.*

Question: What do you give for heparin overdose?
Answer: *Protamine sulfate.*

Question: Patient states, "It is the worst headache of my life," and he has nausea and vomiting; photosensitivity; hypertension; bradycardia; and aphasia. What is the most likely diagnosis?
Answer: *Ruptured cerebral aneurysm.*

Question: What are the guidelines for administering nitroprusside for hypertension?
Answer: *Protect from light with provided covering. Initial dose: 0.3 to a maximum of 10 mcg/kg/min.*

SEIZURES

A seizure is a sudden interruption of electrical brain activity, followed by a postictal state. Many different types are listed here, but the treatment is always the same.

- *Causes:* Aside from febrile seizures, the cause is not always known. Underlying conditions include brain tumor; cerebral infarct; head trauma; medication overdose; and alcohol abuse.
- *Signs and symptoms:* Each type of seizure, with specific signs and symptoms, is listed as follows:
    - *Generalized absence seizure (petit mal):* Characterized by staring or eyelid fluttering for 5 to 10 seconds.
    - *Tonic clonic (grand mal):* Generalized stiffening of extremities, followed by jerking movements; sweating; frothing at the mouth; incontinence; and amnesia.
    - *Partial (focal):* Affects only part of the brain. Symptoms vary according to location of the seizure. It is usually accompanied by an aura. Focal seizures may be the result of underlying problems (e.g., trauma, tumor, or infarct).
    - *Focal motor:* Starts with focal jerking that may persist or may spread to the entire body (grand mal).
    - *Febrile:* Common in infants and young children with high fever.
    - *Status epilepticus:* The seizure that never ends and is therefore an emergency! The patient keeps having one seizure after another, so it looks like one long seizure. The patient with status epilepticus may have increased temperature, BP, and pulse. The patient is at risk for hypoxic brain damage.
    - *Pseudo-seizures:* When the patient is faking a seizure. Yes, this does actually happen! Patient movements may be purposeful, but the patient is not postictal after a fake seizure. This type of seizure is usually preceded by emotional upset and generally lasts longer than a true seizure, and the patient shows stable vital signs.
        - *Arm Test:* Hold the patient's arm above their face, and let go. A truly unconscious patient will hit their face with the arm. The patient with pseudo-seizures will avoid hitting the face.
        - Wave ammonia in front of the patient. If it is a pseudo-seizure, the patient will suddenly be alert and oriented to person, place, and time.

- *Interventions:* Protect the patient from harm but do not restrain; protect airway; place in recovery position afterward; administer oxygen; anticipate orders to obtain an IV access, give medications (lorazepam, diazepam, and anticonvulsants), and reorient to reality after postictal state.

Notes: ____

____

____

____

____

____

____

____

____

____

____

____

Question: How fast do you give IV phenytoin (Dilantin)?
Answer: *Not faster than 50 mg/min to avoid cardiac dysrhythmias and cardiac arrest. In addition, phenytoin (Dilantin) commonly causes phlebitis; be sure to use an in-line filter. If it infiltrates, it causes tissue necrosis!*

Question: Does phenytoin (Dilantin) treat petit mal seizures?
Answer: *No.*

Question: What IV solution can be mixed with phenytoin (Dilantin)?
Answer: *Saline only (think ̲seizure, think ̲saline). Any other solution causes drug to crystallize.*

Question: Do febrile seizures cause permanent brain damage?
Answer: *No.*

Question: What can be mixed with diazepam (Valium) administered intravenously?
Answer: *Absolutely nothing, not even saline, as it will turn chalky.*

BELL'S PALSY

Bell's palsy is paralysis of cranial nerve VII (facial). It usually resolves in several weeks to months.

- *Causes:* Unknown, but it is thought to be caused by a virus or immunodeficiency disorder.
- *Signs and symptoms:* Facial paralysis; headache; facial swelling; numbness; inability to close one eye; facial droop; and drooling.
- *Interventions:* Give medications (steroids, analgesics, artificial tears) as ordered and reassure the patient that they are not having a stroke.

Notes: ____

____

____

____

____

____

____

____

____

____

____

____

____

____

____

____

____

MYASTHENIA GRAVIS

Myasthenia gravis is a neuromuscular disorder.

- *Causes:* Thought to be caused by antibodies inhibiting acetylcholine from transmitting across neuromuscular junction.
- *Signs and symptoms:* Voluntary muscle weakness, especially of the face. Symptoms may improve with rest. Tensilon test is used to diagnose myasthenia gravis, as shown by the significant improvement of the patient after edrophonium is given intravenously.
- *Interventions:* Perform neurologic assessments and give anticholinesterase drugs as ordered.

Notes: ____

____

____

____

____

____

____

____

____

____

____

____

____

____

____

____

____

Question: What is the antidote for anticholinesterase toxicity?
Answer: *Atropine.*

MULTIPLE SCLEROSIS

Multiple sclerosis is a chronic autoimmune disorder in which the body attacks its own myelin sheaths, thereby damaging nerve impulses. The damage affects muscle coordination, strength, sensation, and vision.

- *Causes:* Unknown.
- *Signs and symptoms:* Diplopia; scotomas; tremor; blindness; weakness; fatigue; bladder/bowel incontinence; emotional instability; and paralysis.
- *Interventions:* Anticipate orders to administer diazepam, baclofen, and gabapentin to decrease spasms and tremors.

Notes: ____

CLUSTER HEADACHE

A cluster headache is not one headache but cycles of very painful headaches over 2 to 12 weeks.

- *Causes:* Unknown, but may be attributed to trigeminal nerve dysfunction.
- *Signs and symptoms:* Vary with the individual, but usually include intense pain on one side of the face or eye; runny nose; and nausea and vomiting. Usually, the patient has one tearing, puffy, red eye.
- *Interventions:* Give pain medication and administer 100% oxygen via nonrebreather for 7 to 8 minutes and then rest.

Notes: ____

Table 16.2

Glasgow Coma Scale		
Eye Opening	**Verbal Response**	**Motor Response**
4, spontaneously	5, orientated	6, obeys commands
3, to speech	4, confused	5, localized to pain
2, to pain	3, inappropriate	4, withdraws to pain
1, none	2, incomprehensible	3, flexion to pain
	1, none	2, extension to pain
		1, none

Essential Facts

The Glasgow Coma Scale (Table 16.2) assesses impaired consciousness by evaluating a patient's eye movement, body movement, and verbal responses. A patient with no eye movement, body movement, or verbal response would score a 3.

Contraindications for lumbar puncture include taking warfarin (Coumadin); increased intracranial pressure; intracranial bleed; or infection of the lumbar puncture site.

SUMMARY

You now have a basic knowledge of neurologic emergencies. You should be able to differentiate the various types and know how to treat them. Documenting a patient's complete history and neurologic assessments is absolutely vital. Be familiar with your facility's neurologic assessment tools, such as the NIHSS and Glasgow Coma Scale. **Time is critical to brain tissue; review your hospital's stroke protocol.** Never underestimate your patient's symptoms. Sometimes, a simple headache is the result of cerebral aneurysms, toxins, or brain masses. Therefore, concise assessments and rapid testing are key.

17

OB/GYN Emergencies

Obstetrical (OB) and gynecological (GYN) emergencies occur regularly in the A&E. As a nurse, you must be familiar and comfortable with the various types of OB/GYN emergencies. This chapter guides you through the many common types of OB/GYN challenges, including sexual assault, that you will face in the A&E. When caring for these patients, be sure to always respect your patient's privacy by closing doors and curtains and providing blankets for covering up. Patients may be uncomfortable talking about OB/GYN matters. It is also true that some women are not well educated about their bodies. Some actually do deliver full-term babies in the A&E without knowing they were pregnant. **Thus, the nurse must be sure to document a full and accurate triage and primary and secondary assessment to find the source of the patient's complaint.** You may have to ask a lot of questions to get the necessary patient history. Always be prepared for the possibility and challenges of caring for two patients in one package: mother and baby or babies.

During this part of your orientation, locate and become familiar with:

- Precipitous delivery tray
- Pelvic examination equipment and specimen supplies
- Doppler for fetal heart tones
- Neonatal Apgar documentation
- Local and online Neonatal Resuscitation Program (NRP) Certification

- Facility's policy and procedure for sexual assault, OB in the A&E, methotrexate administration, and RhoGAM administration
- Evidence collection kit
- Medications to know: ceftriaxone (Rocephin), azithromycin (Zithromax), RhoGAM injection, and methotrexate

ENDOMETRIOSIS

Endometriosis is a painful menstrual cycle that occurs because endometrial tissue fragments are found outside the uterus.

- *Causes:* The abnormal tissue fragments react to hormones and slough during menstruation, thereby causing pelvic pain.
- *Signs and symptoms:* Pelvic pain with menstruation; dysuria; irregular menstrual cycles; and abnormal uterine bleeding.
- *Interventions:* As ordered, administer analgesic medication and evaluate effectiveness; order bed rest; set up and assist in pelvic examination; refer patient to OB/GYN specialist.

Notes: ____

____

____

____

____

____

____

____

____

____

____

____

____

____

BARTHOLIN'S CYST

Bartholin's cyst is an obstruction/abscess of the Bartholin gland. The Bartholin gland is responsible for vaginal secretions during sexual arousal.

- *Causes:* Sexually transmitted infection or swelling can cause a clogged or obstructed Bartholin gland.
- *Signs and symptoms:* Pain with intercourse and vaginal lump or abscess.
- *Interventions:* Anticipate orders to administer analgesic/narcotic medications and document effectiveness, prepare for incision and drainage, assist with Word catheter insertion, administer antibiotics, and teach patient about sitz baths.

Notes: ____

____

____

____

____

____

____

____

____

____

____

____

____

____

____

____

____

VAGINITIS

"Vaginitis" is a general term for an altered vaginal flora pH.

- *Causes:* Acquired immunodeficiency syndrome; allergic reaction; bacterial vaginosis; *Trichomonas vaginitis*; foreign object (e.g., old tampon); and yeast (*Candida albicans*) infection.
- *Signs and symptoms:* Red, inflamed vaginal mucosa and abnormal vaginal discharge (see Table 17.1).
- *Interventions:* Prepare for pelvic exam with culture specimen collection as ordered; administer medication according to offending organism; pelvic rest; and patient teaching.

Notes: ____

____

____

____

____

____

____

____

____

____

____

____

Table 17.1

Causes of Vaginitis	
Bacterial Vaginosis	*Candida albicans*
Gray–white, thin, fish-odor vaginal discharge	White, curd cheese–like vaginal discharge
Give metronidazole or clindamycin PO	Give medications fluconazole (Diflucan) PO or miconazole intravaginal

PELVIC INFLAMMATORY DISEASE

Pelvic inflammatory disease (PID) is a vaginal bacterial infection that ascends into and beyond the cervix.

- *Causes:* Usually starts as a vaginal bacterial infection that spreads into and beyond the cervix.
- *Signs and symptoms:* Fever; lower abdominal pain with rebound tenderness; irregular menstrual cycle; foul-odor vaginal discharge; cervical inflammation; "the PID shuffle," shuffling gait due to pain; elevated white blood cell count; and severe pain on pelvic examination.
- *Interventions:* Prepare cultures for pelvic exam; order bed rest; anticipate orders to administer analgesic/narcotic pain medications, evaluate pain medication and document effectiveness, give fluids intravenously or by mouth, administer antibiotics, and teach patient about pelvic rest and prevention.

Notes: ____

____

____

____

____

____

____

____

____

Questions: Which microorganism is the most common cause of PID?

Answer: *Neisseria gonorrhoeae.*

Long-term complications related to under- or untreated PID may include increased risk for ectopic pregnancy and infertility. Discharge instructions should include an emphasis on completion of therapy and follow-up care with gynecologist.

SEXUAL ASSAULT

"Sexual assault" is an assault of a sexual nature on another person, or any sexual act committed against someone's will. It comes in many forms. Most frequently, sexual assaults are committed by a man against a woman. Although less frequent, sexual assault can and does occur to men and children as well.

Rape is the coerced or forced penetration of the vulva or anus with a penis, an object, or any other body part.

The National Sexual Violence Resource Center has a helpful sexual assault toolkit available at www.nsvrc.org/sarts/toolkit/1. It is highly recommended that you take a sexual assault class or become a sexual assault nurse examiner (SANE) to fully understand how to care for the sexually assaulted patient.

- *Causes:* Not all causes are known. However, research shows that sexual assault is sometimes used as an expression of dominance and/or power over the person being assaulted. High-risk behavior of the male perpetrator includes use of drugs or alcohol, lack of inhibitions, history of sexual abuse, sexual promiscuity, associating with sexually aggressive friends, limited economic resources, hostility toward women, and lack of emotional support.
- *Signs and symptoms:* Vary based on the type of sexual assault. Obtaining a good history is critical, as not all sexual assaults will leave visible injuries. Your patient may or may not be tearful and anxious. You may or may not note bruising, lacerations, abrasions, or patterned marks on the patient. Reports of memory loss are not uncommon, and symptoms may indicate the victim is suffering from a toxicologic emergency as well. Be aware of this possibility and implications of drug and alcohol screening in criminal proceedings.
- *Interventions:*
  - Review your facility's policy and procedure for sexual assault.
  - During triage, assess and document the patient's safety and injury, and obtain an accurate, nonjudgmental history in a private location. Use of quotations for subjective data can be helpful. The patient should not wait in the waiting room; triage the sexual assault patient as a higher priority according to the Emergency Severity Index (ESI) handbook.
  - Explain assessments, treatment plans, and options with the patient. These may include prophylactic medications for sexually transmitted infections, pregnancy, and HIV.

- Determine whether the patient wants to file a police report and whether the patient wants evidence to be collected.
- Before you ask the patient to change into a patient gown, remember the clothing the patient is wearing might be evidence. If the clothing was worn during the sexual assault, place two flat sheets on the floor and ask the patient to stand in the middle of the sheet and completely undress. Don gloves to put the underwear in a small **paper bag** labeled "underwear." Do not use plastic bags; they hold moisture that can lead to mold growth, which can damage evidence. Ask the patient to step off the sheet. Then place each item of clothing in separate, small, labeled paper bags. Be sure to change gloves with each item collected, bagged, and labeled. Next, place all bagged and labeled clothing and the top sheet in a large paper bag. Seal, staple, and label the large paper bag with the patient's name.
- Provide privacy and comfort measures such as a blanket, hospital socks, and tissues; allow a friend to stay with patient; and allow normal elimination.
- Perform a complete head-to-toe assessment documenting the injury type, patterned marks, size, shape, number, and location, and whether any penetrating or blunt force trauma occurred. Do not assume anything. Leave your opinions out; document only what you see. Know that your documentation may be used in court.
- If the patient wants evidence to be collected, obtain an evidence collection kit. Be sure to collect everything you need before you open the kit (e.g., pelvic exam equipment, sterile scissors, and sterile water). Once the kit is open and collection begins, you must maintain the chain of custody. Chain-of-custody guidelines require that samples and kits be correctly secured and documented before they can leave your presence. Follow instructions on the kit or according to your facility's policy and procedure. Collections may vary based on type of assault. In general, the order of collection looks something like this:
  - head hair samples
  - oral swabs
  - fingernail cuttings and scrapings
  - other secretions, stains, or forensic material
  - pubic hair samples
  - vaginal/cervical samples (collected by a provider or SANE team member via pelvic exam)
  - anal or rectal samples

Myth: There will always be visible injuries when someone is "really" sexually assaulted.
Reality: Not all sexual encounters cause visible injuries.
Myth: Rape is usually committed by a stranger.
Reality: Most rape victims are raped by a family member or an acquaintance in a private location.

Notes: ____

SEX OR HUMAN TRAFFICKING

Sex or human trafficking is a form of modern-day slavery where a person is bought, sold, and then coerced or forced to perform labor or commercial sexual acts against their will. Roughly 75% of the estimated 40 million global trafficking victims are female (women and girls). Victims may come to the A&E seeking help for injuries or infections; this creates a limited opportunity for nurses to identify and provide a way for them to seek help.

- *Causes:* Sex or human trafficking is the second fastest growing criminal industry and generates billions of dollars. Traffickers prey on society's most vulnerable people with promises of love, relationships, food, fame, drugs, opportunity, and/or money.
- *Signs and symptoms:* School truancy; bruises in various stages of healing; **ownership tattoo or branding mark**; nonlocal or lack of an ID (driver's license); lack of family support; lack of medical care; frequent sexually transmitted infections; drug/alcohol abuse; lice; scabies; frequent mental health problems, such as confusion, fearfulness, anxiety, submissiveness, and withdrawnness; malnourishment; and typically accompanied by another **controlling companion** who coaches them on what to say or speaks for them.
- *Interventions:* Follow your hospital's protocol and state reporting procedures. Nurses are mandated reporters for any suspected minor trafficking victims under 18. Victims are typically reluctant to seek freedom especially if they have had children with their traffickers. They may think you are trying to trap them or test their trafficker's loyalty placing them and their family in danger. **Establish a trusting rapport.** If you suspect human trafficking, **get the victim alone** in a private setting such as the bathroom or radiology or ask companion to leave during assessment. If the victim speaks another language, do not let the companion interpret, use your hospital interpreter. Ask **the victim nonthreatening questions:**
  - Where are you from, how did you get here? Do you know where you are now?
  - Do you keep your own identification papers?
  - Where do you sleep? Is it clean?
  - Do you get enough food to eat?
  - Can you come and go as you please?
  - Are you ever threatened or pressured to work or perform sexual acts?
  - Have you been physically harmed or threatened?
  - Do you keep all the money you earn?

Offer and post available resources such as the **National Human Trafficking Resource Center (NHTRC) phone number** (1-888-3737-888) where patients can see it. This resource can provide food, shelter, childcare, transportation, legal services, medical aid, mental health counseling, health insurance, and education and employment services. If they deny or refuse help, forcing the issue could cause them to flee and/or be fatally harmed by their trafficker, be empathic and nonjudgmental. Consider writing the NHTRC number down on a small piece of paper and placing it under the sole of their shoe, where it cannot be easily detected by their traffickers. This way, when they are ready to leave they can get all the support they need.

Notes: ____

ECTOPIC PREGNANCY

An ectopic pregnancy occurs when a fertilized egg implants any-where outside of the uterus (usually in the fallopian tubes). Compli-cations include a ruptured ectopic pregnancy and hemorrhage.

- *Causes:* The cause is not always known, but PID with scarring and tubal ligation are contributing factors.
- *Signs and symptoms:* **Unilateral severe sharp pelvic pain is a high alert for impending/imminent rupture.** Cramping or minimal pain may occur in the earlier stages. Absent or slight vaginal bleeding; irregular or missed period; positive pregnancy test; positive Kehr's sign; and signs of shock if fallopian tube is ruptured.
- *Interventions:* Anticipate orders to perform pregnancy test, check human chorionic gonadotropin (hCG) level, arrange for bedside point-of-care pelvic ultrasound and/or pelvic/transvaginal ultrasound, start large-bore intravenous access, set up pelvic examination, perform coagulation studies, type and screen blood, determine Rh factor, check frequent vital signs, and prepare for methotrexate administration or surgery.
- *Complication:* Rupture of the fallopian tube may cause bleeding into the pelvic cavity. Occult bleeding may not be obvious; pain is a hallmark sign. This is a surgical emergency, and significant, uncontrolled bleeding **may lead to hypovole-mic shock.**

Notes: ____

____

____

____

____

____

____

____

____

____

SPONTANEOUS ABORTION (MISCARRIAGE)

Miscarriage occurs before the age of viability (20th week of gestation). Table 17.2 shows the various types of miscarriages: complete, incomplete, threatened, inevitable, septic, and missed. Complications include infection and hemorrhage.

Notes: ____

____

____

____

____

____

____

____

____

Question: A 22-year-old female arrives in the A&E complaining of right lower-quadrant abdominal pain. What must be ruled out?
Answer: *Ectopic pregnancy, kidney stones, and appendicitis.*

Note: One saturated pad or tampon = 5 to 15 mL of blood.

RhoGAM may be ordered for Rh-negative women demonstrating signs and symptoms of ectopic pregnancy and/or spontaneous miscarriage. This product helps desensitize the mother's body, when there is possibility of fetal Rh-positive blood mixing with maternal Rh-negative blood. Such mixing of positive and negative blood could cause a hemolytic reaction, similar to mismatched blood transfusions. RhoGAM may be dispensed from pharmacy or lab, depending on your facility's policy. It is important to know the policies, process, and guidelines for administration and documentation at your hospital.

Rachel's Gift (www.rachelsgift.org) and your labor and delivery department are great resources to help provide patients with infant loss and grief support.

Table 17.2

Types of Miscarriages

	Threatened	Complete	Incomplete or Inevitable	Septic	Missed
Symptoms	Slight vaginal bleeding Mild uterine cramps Closed/slightly opened cervix Intrauterine pregnancy on US Fetal heart tones	Slight vaginal bleeding No uterine cramps Closed cervix No intrauterine pregnancy on US All products of conception have passed	Severe vaginal bleeding and clots Moderate uterine cramps Open cervix Ruptured amniotic membranes	Foul vaginal dc/bleeding Severe abdominal/pelvic pain Fever; chills Open cervix	Slight vaginal bleeding Closed cervix No fetal heart beat or intrauterine products of conception noted on US
Interventions	Pelvic exam Pelvic US RhoGAM injection if Rh is negative Bed and pelvic rest[a] OB/GYN follow-up CBC	Pelvic exam Pelvic US RhoGAM injection if Rh is negative Bed and pelvic rest[a] CBC OB/GYN doctor follow-up	Pelvic exam Pelvic US RhoGAM injection if Rh is negative Bed rest CBC Type and screen Pelvic rest[a] OB/GYN follow-up	Pelvic exam/US Blood cultures; CBC IV antibiotics Recheck vital signs RhoGAM injection if Rh is negative Bed and pelvic rest[a] IV fluids and oxytocin Possible D&C OB/GYN follow-up	Pelvic exam Pelvic US Coagulation studies Bed and pelvic rest[a] OB/GYN follow-up Possible surgical intervention

[a]Pelvic rest means no sexual intercourse, no tampons, nothing inside vagina.

CBC, complete blood count; D&C, dilation and curettage; dc, discharge; IV, intravenous; US, ultrasound.

PLACENTA PREVIA

Placenta previa occurs when the placenta implants itself in the lower uterus, thereby partially or completely covering the cervical opening.

- *Causes:* Unknown.
- *Signs and symptoms:* **Painless bright red vaginal bleeding** during pregnancy, and soft nontender abdomen.
- *Interventions:* Anticipate orders to provide bed rest, start large-bore intravenous access, monitor fetal heart tones and frequent vital signs, count menstrual pads, monitor for signs of shock, position the patient on left lateral side, arrange for pelvic ultrasound, type and crossmatch, and complete blood count (CBC). ***Pelvic exam is contraindicated, as it could cause further bleeding.*** **Get the patient to the birth center** and prepare for possible emergency Cesarean section. Remember, "If the bleeding is bright and new, you **cannot** do" the pelvic exam.

Notes: ____

____

____

____

____

____

____

____

____

____

____

____

____

____

____

ABRUPTIO PLACENTAE

Abruptio placentae occurs when the placenta breaks away from the uterine wall before delivery.

- *Causes:* Not always known but can be attributed to abdominal trauma or a very short umbilical cord pulling on the placenta.
- *Signs and symptoms:* Abdominal pain/cramps; profuse or concealed ***dark red vaginal bleeding***; backaches; uterine contractions; fetal distress; and signs of **hemorrhagic shock**. Small concealed bleeds may be asymptomatic.
- *Interventions:* Position patient on her left side; administer high-flow oxygen via nonrebreather mask; monitor fetal heart tones, frequent vital signs, and cardiac rhythm. Anticipate orders to begin large-bore intravenous access; perform coagulation studies; CBC; type and screen blood with Rh; prepare for possible emergency Cesarean section and massive or emergency blood transfusion; and notify and transport to birth center or the operating room.

Notes: ____

____

____

____

____

____

____

____

____

____

Question: What is the major difference between placenta previa and abruptio placentae?

Answer: *Placenta previa has painless bright red vaginal bleeding; abruptio placentae has painful dark red vaginal bleeding.*

PREGNANCY-INDUCED HYPERTENSION OR GESTATIONAL HYPERTENSION

Pregnancy-induced hypertension is diagnosed hypertension that occurs only during pregnancy, usually after the 20th week. **Postpartum patients may suffer from preeclampsia up to 8 weeks after delivery** before the blood pressure is normotensive again. Systemic vasoconstriction may compromise both the placenta and fetal circulation.

PREECLAMPSIA

Preeclampsia is a pregnancy-related complication characterized by gestational hypertension plus proteinuria.

- *Causes:* Unknown.
- *Signs and symptoms:* Hypertension; headaches; edema; epigastric pain; sudden weight gain; **proteinuria**; double vision; uterine contractions; and vaginal bleeding.
  - HELLP (Hemolytic anemia, Elevated Liver enzymes, and Low Platelet count) signs and symptoms: Hypertension, visual changes, headache, nausea, epigastric pain, increased deep tendon reflex, and elevated liver enzymes during the third trimester.
- *Interventions:* Monitor blood pressure; perform urinalysis; arrange for transvaginal or pelvic ultrasound; order bed rest; position patient on left side; monitor urine output; anticipate orders to obtain a complete metabolic panel, a CBC, and a liver function test; monitor cardiac performance and fetal heart tones; begin intravenous access; prepare for possible hospital admission; take seizure precautions; obtain OB consultation; and consider administering intravenous magnesium sulfate. Then prepare for admission or transfer to OB or women's services.

Notes: ____

____

____

____

____

____

____

____

ECLAMPSIA

Eclampsia is a seizure associated with preeclampsia. This is an emergency! During a seizure, circulation of oxygen and nutrients may be compromised to mother and fetus.

- *Causes:* Unknown.
- *Signs and symptoms:* Seizure activity associated with preeclampsia symptoms, including hypertension; headaches; edema; epigastric pain; sudden weight gain; proteinuria; double vision; uterine contractions; decreased fetal heart rate; and vaginal bleeding.
- *Interventions:* Treat airway, breathing, and circulation (ABCs) first and take seizure precautions. Anticipate orders to begin intravenous access; take serum uric acid and liver function tests; perform a CBC and basic metabolic panel; measure hourly urine output; administer anticonvulsants intravenously (e.g., magnesium sulfate); administer hydralazine intramuscularly or intravenously if diastolic blood pressure is >110 mmHg; monitor cardiac performance, level of consciousness, and blood pressure; take seizure precautions; provide psychosocial support; consult with OB; notify labor and delivery units; and prepare for emergent delivery.

Notes: ____

____

____

____

____

____

____

____

____

____

____

____

PROLAPSED CORD

The cord is prolapsed when a pregnant woman comes into the A&E in active labor and you see the cord hanging out. **Get her to the birth center immediately.**

- *Causes:* Unknown.
- *Signs and symptoms:* A woman in active labor with the umbilical cord presenting through the vaginal canal before the baby.
- *Interventions:* Do *not* try to put the cord back in. Manual pressure can be applied to the baby's head by gently pushing up with the finger to relieve pressure on umbilical cord. Manual pressure may need to be maintained until appropriately relieved. Prepare for emergency Cesarean section. Maternal positioning with hips up and head down may help relieve fetal pressure on the cord, but monitor and ensure maternal ABCs are not compromised.

Notes: ____

____

____

____

____

____

____

____

____

____

____

____

____

____

____

____

TRAUMA DURING PREGNANCY

This trauma is the result of an injury that occurred during pregnancy.

- *Causes:* Vary individually. Shift in weight and unsteady gait contribute to falls and injuries during pregnancy. Be alert for the possibility of interpersonal violence.
- *Signs and symptoms:* Vary depending on the injury. May include vaginal bleeding, ruptured membranes, or even **abdominal asymmetry if uterine rupture.**
- *Interventions:* Assess uterine contractions and fetal heart tones (normal is 120–160 beats/min); place the patient in left lateral recumbent position; anticipate orders to obtain large-bore intravenous access; administer isotonic intravenous fluids; determine presence of any amniotic fluids with pH strip; inspect vaginal opening for crowning; check for any fetal movement; palpate and determine fundal height; arrange for pelvic or transvaginal ultrasound and CT scan; perform coagulation studies; prepare a CBC; type and screen blood; arrange for pelvic examination; assess breath sounds for pulmonary edema; prepare for blood transfusion; and prepare for emergency Cesarean section. **No vasopressors** due to fetal compromise.

Notes: ____

____

____

____

____

____

Essential Facts

- If a pregnant patient is on a backboard, tilt the client to her left side to move the uterus off the inferior vena cava.
- Consider early blood transfusion. Large quantities of isotonic fluids do not improve fetal hypoxia.
- A pregnant trauma patient can lose up to 30% of blood volume before becoming hypotensive.

EMERGENCY DELIVERY

It is rare, but sometimes babies are delivered in the A&E. Most times, we feel ill prepared. Sometimes, patients do not know they are pregnant or are in denial. Just remember: Women have been delivering babies naturally without hospitals and nurses since the beginning of time.

- *Causes:* There are only three reasons to deliver a baby in the A&E.
  1. The patient in active labor did not know she was pregnant.
  2. The patient is miscarrying and is less than 20 weeks pregnant.
  3. The active labor patient accidentally comes to the A&E instead of to the birthing center and delivers prior to being transferred to the birthing center.
- *Signs and symptoms:* "Bloody show" or loss of mucus plug; amniotic fluid leakage; frequent contractions; crowning or a visible baby's head; and an uncontrollable desire to push (patient may ask to use the bathroom).
- *Interventions:* Position the patient on her left side; administer oxygen; and visually check for crowning. If signs of imminent delivery are present, be prepared to "catch" the baby; obtain intravenous access as ordered; monitor fetal heart tones and contractions; and prepare for rapid vaginal examination unless vaginal bleeding is present. Vaginal bleeding due to placenta previa may cause life-threatening hemorrhage.
  - *Infant resuscitation:* You have caught the baby; now what? Call for help if you do not have any. You now have two patients, so you need one nurse for the mother and one for the infant.
  - *Prevent heat loss by drying the baby* and wrapping the baby in warm blankets/towels; use warming light; and place baby directly against mother's chest and cover both.
  - *Suctioning:* Bulb suction mouth, then nose. If you do not have bulb suction, use wall suction with oral Yankauer adapter.
  - *Provide oxygen:* If neonatal oxygen levels do not steadily rise above 94% within 10 minutes of delivery (see Table 17.3).
  - *Stimulate:* If the drying and the suction do not work, rub the infant's back or flick/slap soles of feet. If still not breathing, use bag valve mask to assist ventilations.
  - *The Apgar score* is used to determine fetal status. Use Table 17.4 to determine the baby's score. You want the baby to score a perfect 10 by the 10th minute postdelivery.

Notes: ____

Question: Where would a 32-week-pregnant patient diagnosed with appendicitis be hurting?
Answer: *Right upper-quadrant because the appendix gets pushed up later in pregnancy.*

Question: What does "gravida" mean? What does "para" mean?
Answer: *"Gravida" means the number of pregnancies. "Para" means the number of live births.*

The Neonatal Resuscitation Program (NRP) may also benefit the A&E nurse on the assessment, interventions, and specific care needs of infants intra- and postdelivery, and during the neonatal stage of life (0–30 days).

Table 17.3

Target Neonatal Room Air Oxygen Levels Postdelivery	
Time postdelivery	**Pulse oxygen levels**
1 minute	60%–65%
2 minutes	65%–70%
3 minutes	70%–75%
4 minutes	75%–80%
5 minutes	80%–85%
10 minutes	85%–95%

Table 17.4

The Apgar Score			
Sign	**0**	**1**	**2**
Color	Cyanotic/ blue	Body pink, blue extremities	Whole body pink
Muscle tone	Limp	Some flexion	Active movement
Respirations	Absent	Slow, irregular	Good (30–60 bpm)
Heart rate	Absent	Slow (<100 bpm)	Good (100–180 bpm)
Reflex irritability (tactile stimulation)	No response	Facial grimace	Cry, cough, sneeze

POST-BIRTH WARNING SIGNS

Sometimes, postpartum patients show up to the A&E a few weeks after delivery with serious complications, such as hemorrhage, infection, preeclampsia, embolism, or postpartum depression. Document a thorough primary and secondary assessment. Following is the mnemonic **POST BIRTH** to help you remember what to watch out for.

Pain in chest
Obstructed breathing, shortness of breath, or dyspnea
Seizures
Thoughts of hurting self or baby
Bleeding (soak through one pad/hr or egg-sized clots)
Incision that is not healing
Red or swollen leg that is warm and painful to touch
Temperature >100.4 °F
Headache and/or visual changes that don't improve with medications

Notes: ____

SUMMARY

You should now have a more detailed knowledge of OB/GYN emergencies. Be sure to locate and be familiar with all your OB/GYN equipment. Nothing is worse than running around trying to find supplies during an emergency. Be sure to practice assisting with a couple of pelvic examinations during your orientation. At first, you may feel like you need a few extra hands to assist with the examinations. Obtain a good history! This means asking questions, such as when did it start, does anything make the pain worse, and how many pads did you go through today? With pregnant patients, consider the fact that you may have two or more patients. Always be professional and respect your patient's privacy.

18

Ocular Emergencies

You will come across a variety of eye emergencies working in the A&E. Some are as simple as pink eye, whereas others require emergency ophthalmic surgery. **As a nurse, you must be able to differentiate between nonurgent and emergent eye complaints.** This chapter guides you through the various types of eye emergencies and teaches you the manifestations and interventions for each. Be sure to practice with the eye supplies available at your facility during your orientation. Familiarization with your supplies will enable you to obtain a thorough eye assessment of your patients. The providers with whom you work will be expecting a visual acuity test on all eye complaints. **Document carefully and keep your eyes open**—you never know what you will see next in the A&E.

During this part of your orientation, locate and become familiar with:

- Wood's lamp, slit lamp, tono-pen, or tonometer
- Eye exam supplies (fluorescein strips, tetracaine or proparacaine hydrochloride [Alcaine] eye drops and tono-pen covers)
- Visual acuity charts
- pH indicator strips
- Morgan lens and eye irrigation supplies
- Gentamicin ophthalmic ointment
- Eye patches

- All patients with eye complaints need to have their visual acuity documented.
- OS (*oculus sinister*) is left eye. OD (*oculus dexter*) is right eye. OU (*oculus uterque*) is both eyes.

CENTRAL RETINAL ARTERY OCCLUSION

This is a thrombus or embolus central retinal artery occlusion. There is a *1-hour* window to restore blood flow. **This is a true ocular emergency!**

- *Causes:* Just as with a stroke, thrombi or emboli can occlude the retinal artery, cutting off the blood supply to the eye.
- *Signs and symptoms:* Sudden/painless/unilateral/complete loss of vision; dilated nonreactive pupil; and pale fundus.
- *Interventions:* Check the patient's visual acuity; obtain eye exam equipment; anticipate orders to obtain intravenous access, administer vasodilators (e.g., intravenous nitroglycerin) and anticoagulants, arrange ophthalmology consult, and prepare for surgery.

Notes: ____

____

____

____

____

____

____

____

____

____

____

____

____

____

GLAUCOMA

Acute open-angle glaucoma occurs from optic nerve damage.

- *Causes:* It starts with blockage of the outflow of fluid from the anterior chamber. This results in elevated intraocular pressure leading to optic nerve damage.
- *Signs and symptoms:* Diminished vision; deep eye pain; nausea and vomiting; tearing; photophobia; cloudy cornea; semidilated nonreactive pupils; red conjunctiva; and increased ocular pressure.
- *Interventions:* Perform visual acuity test; anticipate provider will monitor ocular pressure; administer myotic eye drops/topical beta antagonists as ordered; and obtain ophthalmologist consult.

Notes: ____

CORNEAL ABRASIONS

These are scratches/abrasions to the clear surface (cornea) of the eye with or without foreign bodies.

- *Causes:* Practically anything that can scratch the skin can scratch the cornea. In most cases, the abrasion is caused by some type of foreign body.
- *Signs and symptoms:* Eye pain; corneal irregularity; no corneal luster; photophobia; copious tearing; and foreign body sensation.
- *Interventions:* Assess visual acuity; obtain eye exam equipment (eye kit, Wood's lamp); anticipate orders to administer antibiotic eye drops or ointment, update tetanus/diphtheria shot, administer oral analgesics, and provide ophthalmologist referral. Research shows that patching may not improve healing or reduce pain, so teach the patient to use "eye rest"—listen and not read or watch screens. Stress the importance of ophthalmologist follow-up.

Notes: ____

____

____

____

____

____

____

____

____

____

____

____

____

____

____

____

DETACHED RETINA

The retina is made of two layers (outer pigmented and inner sensory). A detached retina occurs when these layers separate.

- *Causes:* Vitreous humor leakage; eye trauma; inflammatory disorders; and uncontrolled diabetes.
- *Signs and symptoms:* Painless decreased vision; smoky or cloudy vision; flashing lights; and peripheral floaters (black dots)/"curtain effect."
- *Interventions:* Check visual acuity; position patient supinely; anticipate orders to arrange ophthalmology consult, administer mydriatic drops to dilate pupil, apply bilateral eye patches, and prepare for surgery and admission.

Notes: ____

____

____

____

____

____

____

____

____

____

____

____

____

____

____

____

____

CONJUNCTIVITIS/PINK EYE

This is an inflammation of the conjunctiva. Bacterial and viral conjunctivitis are highly contagious.

- *Causes:* Bacteria, viruses, chemicals, or allergies.
- *Signs and symptoms:* Itchy eyes; photophobia; normal visual acuity; purulent or serous eye discharge; reddened conjunctiva; and copious tearing.
- *Interventions:* Assess visual acuity; anticipate orders to instill topical anesthetic, obtain fluorescein staining supplies and Wood's lamp, and instill ophthalmic antibiotic eye drops or ointment.

Notes: ____

____

____

____

____

____

____

____

____

____

____

____

____

Essential Facts

Because conjunctivitis is so contagious, discharge instructions should include strict handwashing after touching eye area, no sharing of hand towels, discarding current eye makeup, and disinfecting sunglasses.

PENETRATING TRAUMA

Penetrating trauma requires immediate ophthalmology consult. Protruding objects are *not* to be removed but carefully secured in place.

- *Causes:* These vary. You name it, but anything from knives and bullets to nails shot through nail guns have been seen in the A&E. Practically anything with enough force behind it can cause penetrating trauma to the eye.
- *Signs and symptoms:* Irregular pupil shape; impaired visual acuity; and decreased intraocular pressure.
- *Interventions:* Prepare for ophthalmology consult; cover injured eye with metal or plastic patch and patch other eye to reduce eye movement; place patient in semi-Fowler's position; anticipate orders to administer pain medication and give tetanus/diphtheria injection.

Notes: ____

____

____

____

____

____

____

____

____

____

____

____

____

____

BLUNT TRAUMA BLOWOUT FRACTURES

This is a fracture of the orbital floor.

- *Causes:* Inferior orbital rim trauma.
- *Signs and symptoms:* Change in gaze; diplopia; ecchymosis; subconjunctival hemorrhage; paresthesia; periorbital edema; crepitus; and **inability to look up** due to inferior rectus/inferior oblique muscle entrapment.
- *Interventions:* Apply ice pack; anticipate orders to administer pain medications, arrange for orbital x-rays or CT scan, place patient in semi-Fowler's position, and prepare for possible admission or surgery.

Notes: ____

____

____

____

____

____

____

____

____

____

____

____

____

____

____

____

____

HYPHEMA

Hyphema is a hemorrhage into the anterior chamber of the eye that results in corneal blood staining, secondary glaucoma, visual impairment, or loss of an eye.

- *Causes:* Eye trauma.
- *Signs and symptoms:* Blood in anterior chamber of eye; impaired visual acuity; and "seeing red" or floater.
- *Interventions:* Elevate the patient's head of the bed to 60°; gently patch both eyes; anticipate orders to arrange immediate ophthalmology consult, monitor intraocular pressure, and administer mannitol or osmotic diuretic for increased intraocular pressure.

Notes: ____

____

____

____

____

____

____

____

____

____

____

Essential Facts

If a patient presents with blunt trauma to the eye and has brown eyes, always assess the patient from the side to look for a hyphema. It will look like a crescent red moon shape at the base of the cornea.

CHEMICAL BURNS

Chemical burns are the result of contact with *acid* or *alkali* solutions. Alkali chemicals penetrate cells deeper causing more tissue damage and can result in loss of vision. **This is a true eye emergency!**

- *Causes:* Foreign chemical contact with the eye. Severity depends on the pH, concentration, and duration of exposure.
- *Signs and symptoms:* Eye pain; visual disturbances; corneal whitening; copious tearing; surrounding skin irritation; and corneal ulceration.
- *Interventions:* Rinse immediately at a sink or eyewash station. Assess visual acuity; check pH with litmus paper; immediately apply copious amounts of normal saline/lactated Ringer's solution; anticipate orders to maintain continuous irrigation until pH of the eye is 6.9 to 7.2, administer ophthalmic ointment, and arrange ophthalmology referral.

Notes: ____

____

____

____

____

____

____

Essential Facts

Acid burns usually require 30- to 60-minute irrigations. Alkali burns damage tissues more deeply and for longer amounts of time; it may take more than an hour to irrigate. This procedure gets fluid everywhere. You will need to give the patient a gown and a towel and have them lie on the stretcher; place the patient in a slight Trendelenburg position. Then place a basin on the floor at the head of the bed. Finally, place a couple of waterproof bed pads folded like a funnel that drain into a basin on the floor.

SUMMARY

Eye emergencies occur pretty routinely in the A&E. It is vital to recognize which ones are emergent and which ones are nonurgent. Be sure to document pupil size, pupil reaction to light, pupil symmetry, and visual acuity. You should now be more confident in recognizing the symptoms and treatments for the various types of eye emergencies and in treating them. However, you need to practice with the current eye supplies at your facility to truly complete your ocular emergency orientation.

19

Pediatric Emergencies

Children can be some of the most delightful and yet scariest patients you will ever meet. Why scary? For two reasons. First, **children cannot always tell you what is wrong.** So you must assess them well and listen to parents. Although sometimes challenging, **family-centered care is crucial,** and parents generally know when something is wrong with their babies. Second, **children may look okay when they are actually in distress** because they are good at compensating. When they can no longer compensate, they deteriorate rapidly. This is called the "plateau effect." This does not leave the A&E staff with much time to resuscitate them. Therefore, you must treat children aggressively at the early signs of distress, which include tachycardia and increased respirations. Hypotension is a late sign, which is followed by rapid deterioration. You will learn about this extensively during your pediatric advanced life support course. **Pediatric emergency nursing really is a specialty of its own,** but this chapter provides you with some of the basic pediatric emergency nursing tools you will need.

During this part of your orientation, locate and become familiar with:

- Broselow tape and cart/bag
- Where to take a pediatric advanced life support class or emergency nurse pediatric course (ENPC)
- Kilogram–pound conversion
- Pediatric acetaminophen (Tylenol) and ibuprofen (Motrin) doses
- Pediatric vital signs
- Papoose board

- Intraosseous needle, also known as "IO needle," placement and use
- Review Emergency Medical Treatment and Active Labor Act (EMTALA) and hospital policy for consent to treat minors
- Stickers, popsicles, crayons, flashlights, and toys, as these are great for passing time and "bribing"

Essential Facts

When children deteriorate, they generally deteriorate more rapidly than adults.

- Pediatric emergencies account for about 20% to 30% of all A&E visits in United States.
- The majority are seen in nonpediatric A&Es.
- Injuries are the fifth leading cause of death in children younger than 1 year of age, after perinatal conditions, congenital abnormalities, sudden infant death syndrome (SIDS), and heart conditions.

Table 19.1 lists all of the pediatric vital signs according to age group. You will need to know these by heart, so it is a good idea to familiarize yourself with these vital signs during your orientation. Basically, the younger the child, the lower the blood pressure and higher the heart rate and respirations will be.

Essential Facts

Obtain blood pressure in children 4 years of age and older. Do not use the words "blood pressure," as it scares them. Tell them you are going to give their arm a hug with an arm-hugging machine or check their arm muscles.

Table 19.1

Age-Specific Normal Vital Signs

Age	Newborn	Infant	Toddler	Preschooler	School Age	Adolescent	Adult
Respirations	40–60	30–63	22–37	20–28	18–25	12–20	12–20
Heart rate	90–205	90–180	80–140	65–120	58–115	50–100	60–100
Systolic blood pressure	67–84	72–104	86–106	89–112	97–115	110–131	120

FEVER

In children, a fever is defined as a rectal temperature of 100.4 °F or higher. Infants younger than 3 months of age with fever are at high risk for having a serious bacterial infection, such as sepsis or meningitis. A febrile child without an obvious source of fever requires an extensive evaluation and possible admission.

- *Causes:* Otitis media; pneumonia; viral/bacterial infections; gastroenteritis; bacteremia; meningitis; and upper respiratory infections.
- *Signs and symptoms:* Poor feeding; rectal temperature >100.4 °F; irritability; lethargy; dry mucous membranes; decreased tear production; sunken or bulging fontanel; tachycardia; and tachypnea.
- *Interventions:* Anticipate orders to give antipyretic medications (acetaminophen [Tylenol] = 15 mg/kg, ibuprofen [Motrin] = 10 mg/kg) by mouth or suppository, administer intravenous fluids for dehydration, and monitor temperature.

Notes: ____

____

____

____

____

____

____

____

____

____

____

____

____

Essential Facts

Sepsis workup in infants younger than 3 months of age includes labs, chest x-ray, and lumbar puncture. Remember when positioning patient for a lumbar puncture, there should be no chin to chest, as this might occlude the airway. Instead, curve shoulders (not the head) forward.

- Fluids after a lumbar puncture may prevent headache in a young child.
- Children's ibuprofen (Motrin) is not given to children younger than 6 months of age.
- A 4-year-old patient with gastroenteritis who is discharged from the A&E should be encouraged to drink small sips of clear liquids as much as they can tolerate to make up fluid loss. Popsicles and Jell-O are kid-friendly choices.

Essential Facts

Collecting a throat swab can be tricky on a toddler or small child. Here are some tips.

- Have child tilt their head back to get better view.
- Say we are going to "tickle your tonsils with this soft q-tip, now stick out your tongue and say ahhh."
- If they won't open their mouths, get holding help. Slide the q-tip gently through their closed lips. Gently advance until you touch their gag reflex. Then their mouth will open to gag for a few seconds. Now you can see the tonsils, swab each one quickly.

EPIGLOTTITIS

Epiglottitis is a rapid swelling and inflammation of the epiglottis that can lead to a life-threatening airway obstruction. It commonly occurs in children 2 to 6 years of age.

- *Causes:* Acute bacterial infection of the epiglottis.
- *Signs and symptoms:* Sudden onset (2–4 hours); drooling; dysphagia or refusing to drink; inspiratory stridor (abnormal sound over trachea); respiratory distress; tripod position; muffled voice; hoarseness; high fever; sore throat; and anxiety.
- *Interventions:* Decrease stimulation (**do *not* make them cry**); maintain position of comfort; permit caregiver to stay with child; give oxygen by any method tolerated (blow-by); anticipate orders to prepare for intubation or emergency tracheostomy, start intravenous access after securing airway, and administer antibiotics.

Notes: ____

____

____

____

____

____

____

____

____

____

____

____

____

____

BRONCHIOLITIS

Bronchiolitis is a viral infection of the bronchioles, with increased mucous secretion that results in mucus plugging and air trapping.

- *Causes:* The respiratory syncytial virus. It mostly affects infants younger than 1 year of age.
- *Signs and symptoms:* Cough; runny nose; poor feeding; respiratory distress; pallor; retractions; grunting; nasal flaring; wheezing; apnea spells; and fever.
- *Interventions:* Anticipate orders to arrange for chest x-ray; administer fluids by mouth or intravenously; isolate; give oxygen; use nebulizers; administer racemic epinephrine, ribavirin; place head of bed up; and prepare for admission, if severe.

Notes: ____

____

____

____

____

____

____

____

____

____

____

____

____

____

____

____

CROUP

Croup is inflammation and edema of the vocal cords, trachea, and bronchi. It most commonly affects children from 6 months to 3 years of age at night in late fall to early winter.

- *Causes:* A viral illness.
- *Signs and symptoms:* Barking cough (*like a barking seal*); inspiratory stridor; hoarse voice; respiratory distress; low fever; and tachycardia.
- *Interventions:* Anticipate orders to administer cool-mist oxygen, give fluids by mouth or intravenously, and give steroids and racemic epinephrine.

Notes: ____

____

____

____

____

____

____

____

____

____

____

Essential Facts

Pediatric intramuscular (IM) injection tips

- Do *not* use deltoid.
- Best site is anterolateral thigh.
- Get everything ready (adhesive bandages, alcohol swabs); bring a colleague to help hold the child.
- Due to volume, most antibiotic IM injections must be divided into two shots and given simultaneously.

SHUNTED HYDROCEPHALUS

Hydrocephalus is commonly caused by obstructed cerebrospinal fluid, which leads to a dilated ventricular system. A shunt is inserted to drain the fluid away from the cranium to the peritoneum or the left atria. Ventriculoperitoneal shunts are the most common. A child might present to the A&E as a result of infection or malfunction of the shunt.

- *Causes:* Obstruction to flow of cerebrospinal fluid.
- *Signs and symptoms:* Fever; behavioral changes; erythema or fluid along shunt tubing track; meningeal signs; acute abdominal pain; diarrhea; peritonitis; increased intracranial pressure; seizure activity; and headache.
- *Interventions:* Maintain support of airway, breathing, and circulation (ABCs); elevate head of bed up 30°; anticipate orders to administer intravenous fluids (often fluid is restricted), diuretics, analgesics, anticonvulsants, and antibiotics and monitor their effectiveness; anticipate need of removal of cerebrospinal fluid from shunt; take seizure precautions; and monitor cardiac performance, respiratory rate, and continuous pulse oximetry.

Notes: ____

____

____

____

____

____

____

____

____

____

____

CHILD MALTREATMENT

Remember that child maltreatment includes physical, emotional, psychological, and sexual abuse, as well as neglect.

- *Causes:* Many nurses find it impossible to understand what causes a person to harm a child, but it can happen in any socioeconomic class and is usually brought on by the adult's inability to cope with stress.
- *Signs and symptoms:* Bruises or fractures in various stages of healing; burn patterns from cigarettes or hot water; human bite marks; head injuries from direct blows or vigorous shaking, alopecia, lip bruising or laceration; loss of teeth; hyphema; corneal abrasion; retinal hemorrhage; orbital fracture; periorbital hematoma; spiral fractures from twisting injuries; and abdominal trauma (abdominal distention, nausea and vomiting, and abdominal pain).
  - A history may provide vital clues. Always interview parents individually, and, if possible, the child separately.
    - Is there any preexisting medical condition that explains present injuries?
    - Does caregiver's history match the mechanism of injury?
    - Does caregiver deny knowledge of injury occurrence?
    - Are there any inconsistent history changes?
    - Was there any delay in seeking medical attention?
    - Is there any history of unexplained suspicious injuries?
    - Has the caregiver bypassed closer medical facilities to reach yours?
    - Is anyone else besides the parents caring for the child?
- *Signs and symptoms of neglect:* Malnourishment; poor hygiene; inappropriate dress; inadequate medical care; bald patches on infant head from being left in crib in one position for long time; abandonment; numerous dental problems; lack of supervision; and educational neglect.
- *Signs and symptoms of sexual abuse:* Genital/rectal trauma; vaginal/rectal bleeding or pain; vaginal discharge; unusual vaginal/rectal dilation; increased rectal pigmentation; dysuria; frequent urination; foreign bodies in vagina/urethra/rectum; pregnancy; difficulty ambulating; sexually transmitted diseases; and bowel incontinence.
- *Interventions:* Anticipate orders to perform labs (HIV, rapid plasma reagin, amylase, and lipase); arrange for CT scan, ultrasound, and x-rays (complete skeletal survey in child younger

than 2 years of age); provide safe environment; treat injuries; provide emotional support to caregiver and child; remain nonjudgmental; explain tests and procedures; allow caregiver to remain with child except during interview; refer to social services; report all suspected cases to child protective services; complete appropriate paperwork; carefully document shape, size, location, and appearance of all injuries; and document reports from caregiver and child word for word in quotation marks. For suspected sexual abuse, lab protocol may include collecting vaginal/cervical/rectal culture; vaginal/rectal fluids; pregnancy test; ABO-antigen typing; and hair specimen.

Notes: ____

____

____

____

____

____

____

Essential Facts

- Parents from any socioeconomic class may be child abusers.
- The abused child does not cry when parent leaves the room.

Question: Which is not considered child abuse?
A. Burns from the ankles down
B. Missing hair on head
C. Belt marks
D. Bruises on bilateral elbows and knees
Answer: *D is correct.*

CONGENITAL HEART DISEASES

There are several different types; they are classified as left-to-right shunts (acyanotic) or right-to-left shunts (cyanotic).

- *Left-to-right shunts (acyanotic)*: Atrial septal defect, atrioventricular septal defect, ventricular septal defect, and patent ductus arteriosus.
- *Right-to-left shunts (cyanotic)*: Tetralogy of Fallot, tricuspid atresia, transposition of the great vessels, aortic stenosis, pulmonic stenosis, and coarctation of the aorta.
- *Causes:* Unknown.
- *Signs and symptoms:* Cyanosis with feeding or activity; decreased urine; edema; cardiomegaly; hepatomegaly; developmental delays; murmurs; tachycardia; bradycardia; tachypnea; dyspnea; cough; respiratory distress; clubbing of fingers or toes; poor peripheral circulation; mottling of extremities; syncope; and "tet spells" (squatting position to relieve dyspnea).
- *Interventions:* Remember the ABCs; provide basic life support if indicated; anticipate orders for arterial blood gas levels, EKG and echocardiogram, and possible cardiac catheter procedure; allow child to be in position of comfort; administer oxygen; use bag valve mask if needed; start intravenous access; set head of bed at 30°; administer medications (digitalis, diuretics, analgesics, and sedatives) as ordered; limit noxious stimuli; and keep comfortably warm.

Notes: ____

____

____

____

____

____

____

____

____

____

NURSEMAID'S ELBOW (RADIAL HEAD SUBLUXATION)

Nursemaid's elbow is a subluxation of the elbow.

- *Causes:* Commonly occurs when a child younger than 5 years of age is grabbed by the forearm to pull up or swing.
- *Signs and symptoms:* No use of suspected arm after pulling mechanism of the forearm. Child may guard arm. No signs of trauma noted.
- *Interventions:* Assist with simple reduction, arrange for x-ray, administer analgesics as ordered, and apply ice pack.

Notes: ____

____

____

____

____

____

____

____

____

____

____

____

____

____

____

____

SUDDEN INFANT DEATH SYNDROME

This is the most common cause of death in infants between 1 month and 1 year of age.

- *Causes:* Unknown. Studies show that placing an infant on their back to sleep helps reduce the risk of SIDS.
- *Signs and symptoms:* Most caregivers report finding an infant in a crib not breathing or face down in crib. Autopsy fails to reveal cause of death.
- *Interventions:* Attempt to resuscitate using pediatric advanced life support protocol, unless obvious rigor mortis has set in. *Refer parents to the SIDS support group.*

Notes: ____

____

____

____

____

____

____

____

____

____

____

____

____

____

____

____

INTUSSUSCEPTION

Intussusception occurs when a segment of the intestines folds over on itself like a telescope. It most commonly occurs in children younger than 1 year of age. Intussusception can lead to obstruction, edema, and bowel necrosis.

- *Causes:* Unknown; although existing medical conditions may be factors.
- *Signs and symptoms:* Change in eating or bowel pattern; colic; crying; drawing up knees; vomiting; currant-jelly–like red stool; recent infection; and palpable sausage-like mass.
- *Interventions:* Anticipate orders to use nasogastric tube for decompression, administer intravenous fluids, give antibiotics, and prepare for surgical reduction if needed.

Notes: ____

____

____

____

____

____

____

____

____

____

____

____

Essential Facts

- After visiting her grandfather, who has shingles, a little girl develops a rash. The rash is most likely chickenpox.

INTRAOSSEOUS INJECTION SITES

Figure 19.1 shows the primary pediatric and adult intraosseous (IO) injection site. Figure 19.2 shows a secondary IO injection site. Consider IO access if intravenous access is unobtainable after attempting for 30 seconds during an emergency situation.

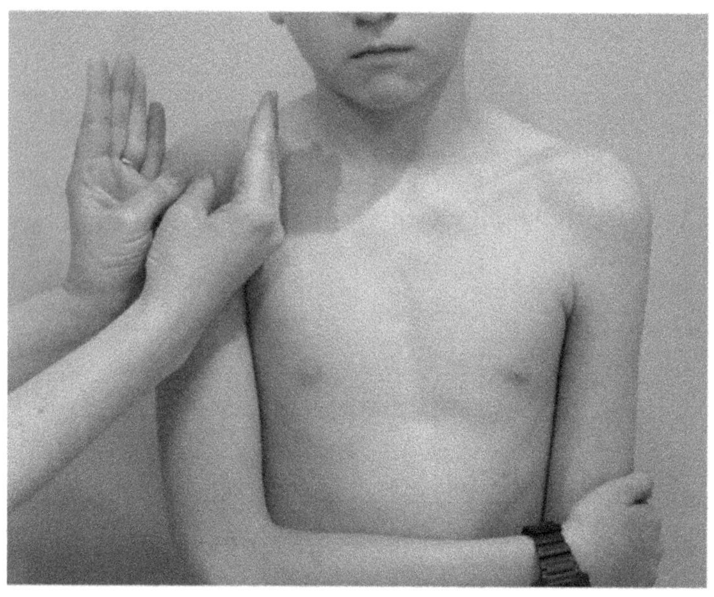

Figure 19.1 Humeral head: Primary pediatric and adult intraosseous site location.

Notes: ____

____

____

____

____

____

____

____

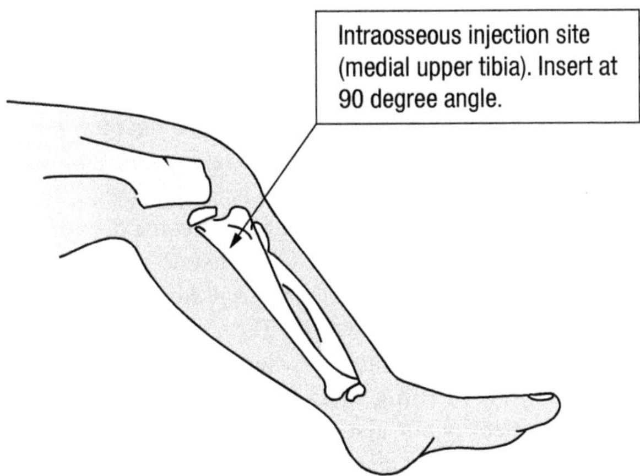

Figure 19.2 Proximal medial tibia: Secondary pediatric intraosseous site location.

Notes: ____

____

____

____

____

____

____

____

____

____

____

____

____

____

____

____

SUMMARY

Pediatric emergency nursing is its own specialty. For the general emergency nurse, the basic information in this chapter will see you through most problems. Be sure to always take account of differences between children and adults. Pediatric patients have different vital signs, deteriorate more rapidly than adults, become dehydrated more easily, and can run higher fevers. All pediatric patient medication doses are based on weight in kilograms. Remember that children cannot always tell you what is wrong. Therefore, it is up to the nurse to obtain an accurate history and detailed physical assessment. If you are ever unsure of something, ask a coworker or go find the answer. The pediatric patient is not just a patient; they are someone's child! Sometimes, the toughest challenge is defusing the hysterical parent's anger or anxiety. Parents do not always realize they are hindering or delaying care when they panic. If the situation cannot be defused, do not waste time. Have another coworker or manager handle the parent, leaving you to care for the child. You now have the knowledge base to diagnose and handle pediatric emergencies. Be careful: These little patients know how to pull on your heart strings.

20

Respiratory Emergencies

Of all emergencies, respiratory problems must be treated first. **Without a patent airway and breathing, your patient will die—and nothing else matters.** Therefore, as an emergency nurse, you must be able to recognize and rapidly respond to any respiratory emergency. This chapter takes you through the most common respiratory conditions seen in the A&E. After reviewing it, you will be able to recognize the various types of respiratory emergencies and know how to intervene.

During this part of your orientation, locate and become familiar with:

- Ambu bags, nasal cannulas, nonrebreather masks, and nebulizers
- Pulse oximetry and waveform capnography devices
- Intubation or cricothyrotomy equipment
- Chest tubes and drainage systems
- Ventilators, bilevel positive airway pressure (BiPAP), and continuous positive airway pressure (C-PAP)
- Reading arterial blood gases (ABGs)
- Medications to know: methylprednisolone sodium succinate (Solu-Medrol), dexamethasone (Decadron), levofloxacin (Levaquin), magnesium sulfate, albuterol, ipratropium bromide (Atrovent), and levobuterol hydrochloride (Xopenex)

Always treat airway first, breathing next, and then circulation. Just remember airway, breathing, and circulation (ABCs).

It is important to recognize when a patient is in respiratory distress or respiratory failure; however, these terms are often misused.

- *Respiratory distress*: results in *decreased* oxygenation and/or ventilation
- *Respiratory failure*: results in *inadequate* oxygenation and/or ventilation

ACUTE RESPIRATORY DISTRESS SYNDROME/ ACUTE LUNG INJURY

Acute respiratory distress syndrome (ARDS) or acute lung injury (ALI) affects children and adults. It is brought about by alveolar histamine release **about 24 to 48 hours after lung injury or illness** resulting in a fluid shift into alveoli and inhibiting surfactant. The result is poor gas exchange, atelectasis, pulmonary edema, hypoxemia, and possible alveolar collapse or fibrosis.

- *Causes:* Near drowning, aspiration, trauma, infection or sepsis, toxins, heroin, cocaine, acute pancreatitis, metabolic disturbances, burns, fat embolism, disseminated intravascular coagulation (DIC), and hematologic disorders.
- *Signs and symptoms:* Severe rapid onset of dyspnea; restlessness; crackles; rhonchi; tachycardia; low pulse oximetry reading despite oxygen therapy; hypoxia; tachypnea; and pulmonary infiltrates on chest x-ray.
- *Interventions:* Anticipate orders to assist ventilations, rapid sequence intubation (RSI); monitor pulse oximetry/waveform capnography; provide high-flow oxygen; obtain intravenous access; obtain portable chest x-ray, ABGs, and serum lactate levels.

Essential Facts

To remember **ARDS**, use the following mnemonic:

Assault to lung tissue
Released histamine
Damaged alveoli
Severe respiratory failure

Notes: ____

____

____

____

____

____

____

____

____

____

____

____

____

____

____

____

____

____

AIRWAY OBSTRUCTIONS

These can be divided into partial, complete, and upper or lower airway obstructions.

- *Causes:* Vary depending on circumstance. Anything from food to coins to a swollen tongue can occlude an airway.
- *Signs and symptoms:* Respiratory distress; dyspnea; choking sensation; drooling; wheezing; decreased or no air movement; aphasia; tachycardia; tachypnea; cough; chest retractions; pallor or cyanosis; and cardiopulmonary arrest.
- *Interventions:* Clear airway; initiate basic life support techniques for foreign-object obstruction; anticipate foreign body removal with Magill forceps by provider and orders to administer oxygen; measure pulse oximetry; if alert and coughing, place in high Fowler's position of comfort; prepare for intubation and possible cricothyrotomy or tracheostomy; document airway patency changes; and document respirations frequently.

Notes: ____

____

____

____

____

____

____

____

____

____

Question: A child swallowed a quarter, is drooling, and has an unusual cough. What is your concern?

Answer: *Airway obstruction (remember your ABCs).*

ASSISTING WITH DRUG-ASSISTED INTUBATION OR RAPID SEQUENCE INTUBATION

Drug-assisted intubation (DAI)/RSI is a technique used to paralyze and sedate an alert or semiconscious patient just prior to performing endotracheal intubation. This process is usually performed by a team including an A&E provider, respiratory therapist, and an advanced cardiovascular life support (ACLS) certified registered A&E nurse.

Rapid Sequence Intubation Preparation Checklist

- Attach cardiac, pulse oximeter, blood pressure, and continuous waveform capnography device to patient.
- Establish intravenous or intraosseous access.
- Provide oxygen supply to patient via nonrebreather mask. Have bag valve mask ready.
- Suction equipment is available and working properly.
- Nasal or oral pharyngeal airways are available in appropriate sizes.
- Endotracheal tubes with stylets are available in appropriate sizes.
- Laryngoscope with curved or straight blades are available and working (and video laryngoscope).
- 10-mL syringe to test inflate endotracheal balloon is available.
- Endotracheal securement device or cloth tape is available.
- Crash cart is in room.
- Rescue or difficult airway equipment is available.

Rapid Sequence Intubation Step by Step

- Prepare equipment (see previous checklist).
- Open airway (maintaining C-spine immobilization if injury present).
- Pre-oxygenate patient with 100% oxygen via nonrebreather or bag valve mask.
- Anticipate orders to premedicate as indicated for increased risk of bradycardia or increased intracranial pressure:
  - *Atropine (Atropen):* Adults: rescue dose; pediatrics: 0.01 to 0.02 mg/kg (max 0.5) to inhibit bradycardia response.
  - *Fentanyl:* Adults: 1 to 3 mcg/kg; pediatrics: 1 mcg/kg to prevent intracranial pressure increase during RSI.
  - *Lidocaine (Xylocaine):* Adults: 100 mg (2% 5-mL syringe); pediatrics: 1.5 mg/kg (max 100 mg) to prevent intracranial pressure and suppress cough reflex during RSI.

- Anticipate orders to administer sedation or anesthesia intravenous (IV) push. Examples are as follows:
  - *Etomidate:* 0.3 mg/kg
  - *Fentanyl citrate (Sublimaze):* 2 to 10 mcg/kg
  - *Ketamine (Ketalar):* 1 to 2 mg/kg. Recommended for asthmatic pediatric intubations.
  - *Midazolam (Versed):* 0.1 to 0.3 mg/kg (max 10 mg)
  - *Propofol (Diprivan):* 1 to 2 mg/kg. Check state law for RN administration conditions
  - *Thiopental (Thiopental):* 2 to 5 mg/kg
- Anticipate orders to administer paralytic or neuromuscular blocking agent IV push. Ensure provider is fully prepared to intubate prior to pushing any of these drugs, as the patient will *stop* breathing once it is given! Examples are as follows:
  - *Succinylcholine (Anectine):* 1 to 1.5 mg/kg. Increases serum potassium and causes bradycardia. **Contraindicated in renal, hyperkalemic, bradycardic, burn, or crush injury patients.** In rare cases, genetic disposition may cause **malignant hyperthermia** after receiving succinylcholine. Monitor for severe high fever, muscle spasms/rigidity, tachycardia, sweating, tachypnea, V-tach/V-fib, and acidosis. Follow your facility's malignant hyperthermia treatment protocol for cooling measures and administration of antidote dantrolene (Ryanodex).
  - *Vecuronium:* 0.1 to 0.2 mg/kg
  - *Rocuronium (Zemuron):* 1 mg/kg
- Provider will assess whether patient is relaxed enough to intubate. Look for jaw relaxation and apnea.
- Monitor continuous pulse oximeter, waveform capnography, and vital signs while provider attempts endotracheal intubation.
- If intubation is successful, provider will inflate balloon. If provider is unsuccessful, be ready to assist ventilations with bag valve mask (1 breath every 6 seconds).
- Confirm placement by attaching bag valve mask to endotracheal tube to listen for bilateral breath sounds; listen to ensure there are no epigastric sounds; attach CO_2 detection device; and monitor waveform capnography.
- Secure endotracheal tube with cloth tape or commercial securement device.
- Document time, confirmed placement methods, endotracheal tube size, and tube placement at the lip. A respiratory therapist will usually attach a ventilator to endotracheal tube at this time.
- *Continue sedation* and frequent vital sign monitoring.

Essential Facts

- When medicating for RSI, always administer sedatives prior to paralytics.
- To troubleshoot any breathing problems after intubation, just use the mnemonic **DOPE**.
    - **D**isplaced tube (right mainstem)
    - **O**bstruction of tube or airway
    - **P**neumothorax
    - **E**sophageal intubation

Notes: ____

____

____

____

____

____

____

____

____

____

____

____

____

____

____

____

____

CHRONIC OBSTRUCTIVE PULMONARY DISEASE

Chronic obstructive pulmonary disease (COPD) is an irreversible chronic obstructive small airway disease. A patient with COPD will have elevated carbon dioxide levels. Over time, the elevated carbon dioxide levels will make the patient dependent on lower PAO_2 level changes (hypoxia) to regulate ventilations. Therefore, if you deliver high-flow oxygen for an extended period of time, the patient will lose their hypoxic respiratory drive *and stop breathing!*

- *Causes:* Enlargement of the alveoli, loss of lung tissue elasticity, and destruction of alveolar wall. This chronic lung damage is associated with emphysema, chronic bronchitis, and cigarette smoking.
- *Signs and symptoms:* Dyspnea; tachypnea; pursed-lip breathing; wheezing; crackles; tripod position; use of accessory muscles; barrel chest; tachycardia; hypertension; confusion; cyanosis; premature ventricular contractions; and acute respiratory failure.
- *Interventions:* Anticipate orders to obtain and monitor ABGs, administer 1 to 2 L of low-flow oxygen because of carbon dioxide retention, position head of bed up 90%, apply BiPAP, give nebulizer treatments and corticosteroids, and give high-flow oxygen via nonrebreather only if the patient is in severe respiratory distress.

Notes: ____

____

____

____

____

____

____

____

____

____

____

____

ASTHMA

Asthma is a reversible chronic reactive airway disease. It is a complex inflammatory response characterized by large airway inflammation and structural changes. Asthma is classified into four categories. Decrease in oxygen level is a late sign.

- *Causes:* A hypersensitive immune system reaction that causes the airways to inflame and swell when exposed to certain triggers. The triggers vary from person to person, but common triggers include dust, pollen, pet dander, exercise, cigarette smoke, medications (aspirin or NSAIDs [nonsteroidal antiinflammatory drugs]), upper respiratory infections, and gastroesophageal reflux disease.
- *Signs and symptoms:* Vary by category.
  - *Mild intermittent:* Expiratory wheezing; pulse oximeter reading of 95% to 100%; and cough.
  - *Mild persistent:* Inspiratory and expiratory wheezing; pulse oxygen of 95% to 100%; and cough.
  - *Moderate persistent:* Inspiratory wheezing; expirations diminished; cough; use of accessory muscles; retractions; nasal flaring; and tripod position.
  - *Severe persistent:* Expirations and inspirations diminished (silent lung); no breath sounds; diaphoresis; dusky pallor or cyanotic skin color; pulse oxygen reading of <95%; bradypnea or periods of apnea; and drowsiness or altered mental status.
- *Interventions:* Anticipate orders to position for comfort; give oxygen, apply pulse oximetry, monitor end-title CO_2, and apply BiPAP or intubate in late stages. For asthma medication orders, **just remember ASTHMA: A**lbuterol, **S**teroids, **T**heophylline **H**ydration, **M**agnesium, and **A**ntibiotics (if infection).

Notes: ____

____

____

____

____

____

____

STATUS ASTHMATICUS

Status asthmaticus is a rare severe asthma exacerbation that doesn't respond to therapy. Mortality rate is significantly high.

- *Causes:* Untreated asthma or rapid severe onset of asthma. History may reveal previous intubations.
- *Signs and symptoms:* Absent breath sounds (silent lung), inability to speak in full sentences or lay flat, pulse oxygen level <90% with supplemental oxygen, altered level of consciousness, fatigue, long expiratory phase, tachypnea with accessory muscle use, and cyanosis. Waveform capnography may reveal "shark fin"–shaped waveform with elevated CO_2 levels due to air trapping.
- *Interventions:* Treat immediately and aggressively with high-flow oxygen, IV magnesium, BiPAP, or intubation. Ketamine is recommended for sedation with asthmatic intubation. Apply pulse oximetry and end-title capnography device. Consider intramuscular (IM) or IV epinephrine and extracorporeal membrane oxygenation (ECMO).

Notes: ____

____

____

____

____

____

____

Essential Facts

As bronchospasms improve or reverse, breath sounds go from diminished to louder to clear.

- Diphenhydramine hydrochloride (Benadryl), propranolol (Inderal), or morphine sulfate may be contraindicated in asthmatic patients. Benadryl can dry and thicken mucus. Inderal can block bronchodilation. Morphine can cause respiratory depression.
- The optimal peak expiratory flow rate is >80% of predicted or personal best.

SPONTANEOUS PNEUMOTHORAX

Spontaneous pneumothorax is an air leak in the pleural space that results in partial or total collapse of the lung.

- *Causes:* Not always known. However, COPD, asthma, cystic fibrosis, tuberculosis, pneumonia, lung cancer, interstitial lung disease, inhaled substance abuse, barometric pressure changes (scuba divers, pilots), ingestion of toxic drug pentamidine, smoking, and immunodeficiency disease all attribute to spontaneous pneumothoraxes.
- *Signs and symptoms:* Dyspnea; tachypnea; tachycardia; sudden pleuritic chest pain; anxiety; restlessness; diminished or absent breath sounds on affected side; pallor; hypotension (if severe); subcutaneous emphysema; palpitations; or asymptomatic (if small).
- *Interventions:* Place in high Fowler's position; prepare for needle thoracostomy, Heimlich valve, or chest tube insertion; and administer pain meds as ordered.

Notes: ____

____

____

____

____

____

____

____

____

____

Essential Facts

If a tall, thin young adult states, "I suddenly coughed and became short of breath," think spontaneous pneumothorax.

BRONCHITIS

Bronchitis is an infection of bronchi.

- *Causes:* Viral or bacterial infection.
- *Signs and symptoms:* Productive cough, crackles, wheezing, fever, pleuritic chest pain, dyspnea, hoarseness, and malaise.
- *Interventions:* Rest, bronchodilators, expectorants, increase in fluid intake, antibiotic, and antipyretics.

Notes: _______________________________________

PNEUMONIA

Pneumonia is an acute inflammatory reaction that results in fluid and cellular debris accumulating in segments and lobes of the lung.

- *Causes:* Aspiration, bacterial, mycoplasmas, fungi, foreign material, protozoan, or viral infections.
- *Signs and symptoms:* Productive cough; green, bloody, or rust color sputum; fever (acute onset); chills; pleuritic chest pain; dyspnea; tachypnea; respiratory distress; tachycardia; confusion; altered level of consciousness; crackles; wheezing; diminished breath sounds; and weight loss.
- *Interventions:* Anticipate orders to obtain intravenous access; obtain blood cultures; administer antibiotics; rehydrate; use nebulizers; monitor pulse oximetry or waveform capnography; give oxygen; order complete blood count and chest x-ray; and give antipyretics (if fever).

Notes: ____

____

____

____

____

____

____

____

____

____

____

____

Question: What is the major pulmonary cause of septic shock?
Answer: *Acute bacterial pneumonia.*

BURN INHALATION

If a patient has burns to the face, consider the possibility of burns to the large and small airways. Patients may appear stable initially but remember that burns swell quickly, resulting in rapid loss of airway.

- *Causes:* Burns to face, neck, chest, mouth, or airway.
- *Signs and symptoms:* Black-tinged sputum; dry mucous membranes; rales; rhonchi; and dry nonproductive cough. Singed nasal hair, eyebrows, and eye lashes.
- *Interventions:* Prepare for emergent intubation, apply nonrebreather oxygen mask, and anticipate order to obtain ABGs.

Notes: ____

SUMMARY

You now have a strong foundation to assess and treat respiratory emergencies. Be sure to thoroughly document respiratory assessments. This should include rate, depth, breath sounds, symmetry, skin color, use of accessory muscles (if labored or unlabored), and ability to speak in full sentences before and after each intervention. It is imperative that you are competent in recognizing and treating all respiratory emergencies. To make you more comfortable with respiratory problems, be sure to familiarize yourself with all your facility's respiratory supplies and equipment. Knowing where your supplies are and how to use them will make your job easier. If you have a lot of questions, a respiratory therapist can be a good resource. Never forget: In any emergency, treat the airway first, then breathing, and then circulation.

21

Shock Emergencies

Patients in shock are considered critical, so a knowledge of these emergencies is vital for the A&E nurse. The window of opportunity to save these patients' lives is small. In this chapter, you will learn the various forms of shock and how to intervene. Be sure to learn your facility's shock protocols and be familiar with shock supplies in your department.

During this part of your orientation, locate and become familiar with:

- Rapid infusers, pressure bags
- Mass and uncrossmatched blood transfusion protocols
- Blood warmers, blood tubing, and blood bank
- Auto-transfuser
- Protocols for sepsis
- Pericardiocentesis tray
- Therapeutic hypothermia policies and protocols
- Anaphylactic drug supply box
- Tourniquet application (military grade)
- Medications to know: dopamine, norepinephrine (Levophed), epinephrine, dobutamine, milrinone, phenylephrine, vasopressin methylprednisolone sodium succinate (Solu-Medrol), dexamethasone (Decadron), diphenhydramine hydrochloride (Benadryl), and famotidine (Pepcid)

SHOCK

Remember that shock simply means "inadequate tissue perfusion," despite the cause. **Early recognition** is the key to reduce mortality and morbidity.

There are three stages to any form of shock.

- *Compensated:* This is the early phase of shock in which the body compensates for the decreased tissue perfusion with vasoconstriction, **mild tachycardia**, decreased urine output, and **tachypnea**, as blood pressure remains **normotensive**, with a slight rise in diastolic blood pressure, resulting in **narrowing pulse pressure. Early recognition and interventions during this phase can improve mortality rates by about 70%.**
- *Decompensated or progressive:* This stage is marked by increased tachycardia, tachypnea, signs of poor circulation, and **hypotension** with a decrease in systolic blood pressure further narrowing the pulse pressure. The body can no longer compensate to maintain adequate tissue perfusion and blood pressure, resulting in metabolic acidosis and elevated lactic acid levels.
- *Irreversible or refractory:* This stage is marked by symptoms of cellular, tissue, and organ or multiorgan death and dysfunction. The patient may have bradycardia, bradypnea, severe acidosis, pallor, petechiae, purpura, severe hypotension, and may be unresponsive. Poor patient outcomes and death are common despite aggressive treatments and interventions.

There are four types of shock:

- Hypovolemic—loss of volume (most common)
  - Hemorrhagic
  - Nonhemorrhagic (dehydration)
- Cardiogenic—pump problem
- Obstructive
  - Cardiac tamponade
  - Tension pneumothorax
  - Massive pulmonary embolism
  - Ductal-dependent congenital heart lesions (obstructs flow from left side to aorta)
- Distributive
  - Anaphylactic
  - Septic
  - Neurogenic

Hypovolemic Shock

This is a decrease in circulating volume. Hypovolemic shock is the most common form of shock in a trauma patient. **Control any external hemorrhage;** hemorrhage is one of the most preventable causes of death.

- *Causes:* Lack blood volume because of laceration of a major blood vessel; gastrointestinal bleeding; severe dehydration; ruptured organ; severe burns; crush injuries; bleeding aneurysm; and poor clotting factors.
- *Signs and symptoms:* Hypotension; **narrowing pulse pressure;** tachycardia; and altered level of consciousness. Early signs and symptoms may include restlessness, anxiety, and confusion.
- *Interventions:* Assess and treat any external hemorrhage, then treat airway, breathing, and circulation (ABCs); monitor vital signs, cardiac performance, and oxygen levels; anticipate orders to obtain two large-bore intravenous (IV) accesses, administer warmed IV crystalloid fluid infusion of 20 to 40 mL/kg, prepare transfusion of whole or packed red blood cells and fresh frozen plasma or platelets, and apply direct pressure or tourniquet to profusely bleeding lacerations. Consider tranexamic acid administration and Resuscitative Endovascular Balloon Occlusion (REBOA).

Notes: ____

____

____

____

____

Essential Facts

When administering **massive blood transfusions,** follow your hospital policy and monitor your patient's **calcium levels** frequently. The preservative in blood products called citrate binds with calcium causing the patient's serum calcium to drop. Calcium is a vital part of the clotting cascade, without which your patient could bleed out even faster despite your all massive blood transfusions.

Question: In a pediatric patient, what are some late signs of hypo-volemic shock?
Answer: *Bradycardia and hypotension. Cyanosis and tachycardia are early signs.*

Question: A patient with hyperosmolar hyperglycemic nonketotic syndrome is at risk for what type of shock?
Answer: *Hypovolemic shock.*

Question: What is the only IV fluid that can be infused with blood?
Answer: *Normal saline.*

Cardiogenic Shock

In cardiogenic shock, the heart fails to pump blood effectively.

- *Causes:* Myocardial infarction; dysrhythmias; cardiac failure; blunt cardiac trauma; or myocardial contusion.
- *Signs and symptoms:* Hypoxia; anxiety; diaphoretic and rapid weak pulse; dysrhythmias; jugular vein distention (JVD); hypotension; S3 heart sound; pulmonary edema; crackles; and tachypnea.
- *Interventions:* Treat ABCs. Anticipate orders to apply cardiac monitor, open two large-bore IV accesses, administer oxygen, take EKG and pulse oxygen, **administer small IV fluid bolus cautiously** and administer appropriate anti-arrhythmic medications, treat the underlying heart condition, and consider inotropic drips such as dobutamine or milrinone.

Notes: ____

Obstructive Shock: Cardiac Tamponade

This is fluid or blood buildup in pericardial sac surrounding the heart.

- *Causes:* Blunt or penetrating chest trauma.
- *Signs and symptoms:* Penetrating chest wound noted to left third to fifth ribs; dyspnea; facial cyanosis; hypotension; ST-segment elevation in all leads on EKG; chest wall ecchymosis; and elevated venous pressure. **Beck's triad: muffled heart sounds, JVD, and hypotension.** Hamman's crunch: crunching, rasping sound heard with the heartbeat.

- *Interventions:* Anticipate orders to monitor cardiac performance, administer oxygen, open IV access, take EKG, and prepare for emergency pericardiocentesis.

Notes: ____

Question: What autoimmune condition may cause cardiac tamponade?
Answer: *Systemic lupus erythematosus.*

Obstructive Shock: Tension Pneumothorax

Tension pneumothorax is a life-threatening complication of pneumothorax.

- *Causes:* The lung totally collapses, and the heart and chest contents actually shift toward the unaffected lung. Blood flow through the aorta is obstructed as thoracic organs shift to one side.
- *Signs and symptoms:* Tracheal shift; severe respiratory distress; hypotension and JVD; dyspnea; tachypnea; tachycardia; sudden pleuritic chest pain; anxiety; restlessness; asymmetrical chest expansion; diminished or absent breath sounds on affected side; pallor; hypotension if severe; subcutaneous emphysema; and palpitations.
- *Interventions:* Treat ABCs; place in high Fowler's position; anticipate orders to prepare for needle thoracentesis and/or chest tube insertion, administer pain medications, arrange for chest x-ray, and apply sterile nonporous dressing (Vaseline gauze) with tape on three sides over an open, penetrating chest wound.

Notes: ____

Question: When a 27-year-old female arrives in the A&E complaining of sudden onset of shortness of breath, what question should you ask?
Answer: *"Are you currently taking any birth control medication?"*

Obstructive Shock: Pulmonary Embolus

Pulmonary embolus is a complete or partial thrombus blockage of the pulmonary artery that results in systemic hypoxia.

- *Causes:* Blood clots or air, fat, or amniotic fluid emboli. Risk factors may include history of thrombus or embolism formation, recent surgery, recent travel, estrogen therapy, cancer, postpartum, smoking, and prolonged immobilization.
- *Signs and symptoms:* Sudden dyspnea and tachypnea; respiratory distress; anxiety; restlessness; confusion; chest pain; cough; hemoptysis; wheezing; diaphoresis; pallor from the nipple line up; fever; hypotension; right-sided congestive heart failure, peaked P waves, right bundle branch block (RBBB), and ST-segment and T-wave changes on EKG; JVD; cyanosis; and respiratory arrest.
- *Interventions:* Anticipate orders to give oxygen; obtain pulmonary angiography or pulmonary ventilation/perfusion scan, spiral CT scan; apply bilevel positive airway pressure; use bag valve mask for ventilatory assistance; prepare for intubation; start IV access; administer IV fluids and anticoagulants; use IV or inhaled bronchodilators; and give analgesics, antidysrhythmics, and thrombolytic and platelet aggregation inhibitor therapy.

Notes: ____

Distributive Anaphylactic Shock

Anaphylactic shock is a systemic antigen–antibody response to an allergic reaction that is associated with sudden severe respiratory distress.

- *Causes:* Unknown, but various triggers may stimulate a severe allergic reaction, including seafood, iodine, certain antibiotics, insect bites, nuts, and various medications or food.
- *Signs and symptoms:* Laryngeal edema; bronchospasms; wheezing; angioedema; and hypotension due to peripheral vasodilation.
- *Interventions:* Establish airway; apply oxygen; monitor cardiac performance; open IV access; obtain anaphylactic drug box; and administer medications (epinephrine, antihistamines, bronchodilators, Pepcid, and IV steroid) as ordered.

Notes: ____

Essential Facts

It is important to understand which concentration of epinephrine to administer for anaphylaxis. You do not want to give the wrong one. As odd as it sounds, an easy way to remember the difference is to compare them to a tequila shot and a margarita. Both drinks have tequila in them, but one is diluted, and one is concentrated. Epinephrine also comes in concentrated forms and a diluted form.

- Epinephrine 1:1,000 comes in a 1 mg/1 ml ampule/vial and is concentrated like a shot of tequila and therefore can be given only subcutaneously or intramuscularly (SQ/IM) for anaphylaxis.
- Epinephrine 1:10,000 comes in a large premixed syringe (1 mg/10 ml) and is diluted like a margarita. Therefore, it can be given intravenously, typically during cardiopulmonary arrest.

Distributive Septic Shock

This is a systemic infection or severe sepsis with poor profusion despite adequate fluid resuscitation. The very young, elderly, and immunosuppressed patients are more at risk. It can lead to **systemic inflammatory response syndrome (SIRS).**

- *Causes:* Typically, due to gram-negative or gram-positive bacteria. The infection usually stems from one source and then spreads to the rest of the body through the bloodstream. A massive SIRS is launched by the body, which results in vasodilation and hypotension.
- *Signs and symptoms:* Fever, flushed skin, bounding pulses, vasodilation, tachycardia, widening pulse pressure, and anxiety are noted in early (warm) stages. Hypothermia, tachypnea, hypotension, pallor, mottled skin, scant urine output, increased lactic acid, weakness, and coma are noted in late (cold) stages.
- *Interventions:* Look for underlying infection; monitor vital signs and temperature; and anticipate orders to start IV access and fluid bolus of 30 mL/kg (caution if renal failure or congestive heart failure). Obtain blood cultures, complete blood count, procalcitonin, and **lactic acid levels**; administer IV antibiotics; and obtain urine culture.

Notes: ____

SIRS criteria: Two or more of the following symptoms may be indicative of sepsis:

- Temperature >38 °C (100.4 °F) or <36 °C (96.8 °F)
- Heart rate >90 beats per minute
- Respiration rate >20 breaths per minute, or hyperventilation and PaCO$_2$ <32 mmHg
- White blood cell (WBC) count >12,000 mm^3, <4,000 mm^3, or >10% immature neutrophils (bands)

Question: Would you obtain blood cultures before or after administering IV antibiotics?

Answer: *Before. Take cultures from two different sites.*

Distributive Neurogenic Shock

This is the loss of sympathetic vasomotor regulation.

- *Causes:* Brain stem injury, spinal anesthesia, or spinal cord injury. Other causes may include drug use, such as tranquilizers, barbiturates, or anesthetics.
- *Signs and symptoms:* Peripheral vasodilation; neurologic deficits; **bradycardia**, respiratory depression, paraplegia/quadriplegia, priapism, poikilothermia, warm or flushed skin; and severe hypotension.
- *Interventions:* Provide ABCs; maintain cervical (C-spine) immobilization if spinal cord injury is present. Anticipate orders to obtain IV access; administer IV fluid bolus; make neurologic assessments; give dopamine or norepinephrine (Levophed), atropine for symptomatic bradycardia; maintain normal temperature; and reduce intracranial pressure.

Notes: ____

SUMMARY

After reading this chapter, you should now have a stronger knowledge base for shock-related emergencies. You should be able to differentiate among the various types of shock. Although all shocks result in inadequate tissue perfusion, each type of shock has a completely different cause. You must identify the cause to implement the right treatment course. **Mortality rates are drastically improved by identifying and treating *early stages of shock*.** Be observant for those subtle vital sign changes found in the early signs of shock. Early rapid responses save lives and preserve end organs.

22

Substance Abuse and Toxicologic Emergencies

Substance abuse and toxicologic conditions, which are seen regularly in the A&E, can be fatal. From 1999 to 2017, 700,000 additional lives have been lost to drug overdose. The death rate related to drug overdose has risen incrementally by the tens of thousands year over year for the last decade. Because so many types of substance abuse and poisonous materials exist, remembering them all is difficult. Increasingly, teenagers and young adults are vaping various substances and finding creative inexpensive ways to get high. These may include **synthetic drugs** or household substances such as nutmeg, poisonous flowers, cough syrups, and taking family members' prescribed home medications. A detailed assessment and **patient history are key** to identifying the substance taken. Be sure to include feedback from any witnesses, friends, or family who may be willing to disclose what was taken. This chapter provides a simple and easy-to-use substance abuse and toxicology table. Even with access to this table, you must still **always consult with poison control** after the patient is triaged. Poison control will give you vital individualized suggestions based on the patient's weight, circumstances, amount of drug intake, and the time frame in which the drug was taken. Document and communicate the suggestions provided by poison control with the A&E provider to obtain any necessary immediate orders.

Many controlled substances are being inhaled via electronic cigarette or vaping devices. These vaping devices can be disguised as other small objects such as plug or outlet connections, or universal serial bus (USB) devices. See Figure 22.1 for various types of vaping devices.

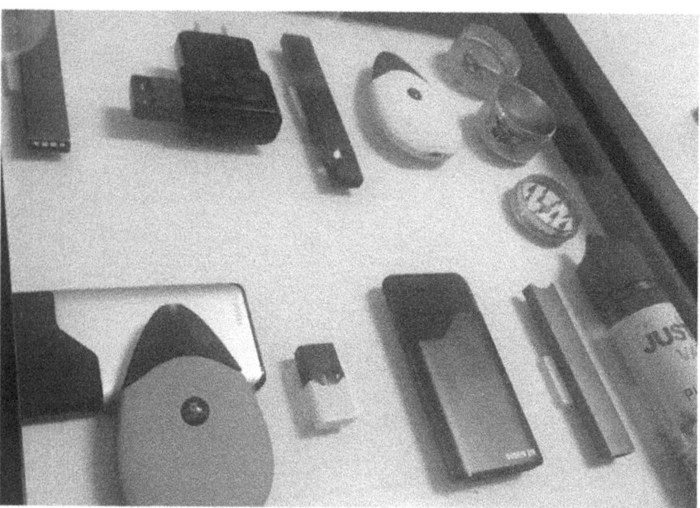

Figure 22.1 Different types of vaping devices.

During this part of your orientation, locate and become familiar with:

- Local poison control number
- Your local poisonous snakes and appropriate antivenom information
- Nasogastric tubes and gastric lavage equipment
- Medications to know: charcoal with or without sorbitol, naloxone (Narcan), flumazenil (Romazicon), acetylcysteine (Mucomyst), and banana bag (various institution-specific formulations, for example, intravenous [IV] fluids containing folic acid, thiamine, and multivitamin).

Essential Facts

- Call poison control for **every** overdose.
- Treatment of most overdose patients generally begins with the **ABCs** (**A**irway, **B**reathing, and **C**irculation) and **MOVE** (**M**onitor, **O**xygen, **V**enous access, and **E**KG).

Table 22.1 is a great quick reference tool to assist you with substance abuse and toxicology cases. In it, you will find an alphabetical list of each substance or drug class, with the corresponding drug-effect symptoms and interventions. Examples of drugs and substances are provided under each class.

Question: Why can't you rely on a pulse oxygen reading in carbon monoxide poisoning?

Answer: *Carbon dioxide, ethane, methane, propane, and other fuel gases bind to hemoglobin, preventing oxygen from binding to the hemoglobin. Therefore, you cannot rely on a pulse oxygen reading. Treatment is "fresh air" or supplemental oxygen.*

Question: Ecstasy use along with increased water intake to avoid hyperthermia can lead to what electrolyte imbalance?

Answer: *Hyponatremia.*

Question: A college student arrives in the A&E complaining of palpitations and chest pain. He admits to using cocaine. What should you suspect?

Answer: *Acute myocardial infarction.*

Question: How does charcoal leave the digestive system?

Answer: *Usually it comes out in the form of black diarrhea. An unconscious or confused patient may need an incontinence pad.*

Notes: ____

Table 22.1

Substance Abuse and Toxicology Table

Drug/Substance	Signs and Symptoms	Interventions/Anticipated Orders
Acetylcholinesterase inhibition (cholinergics) Insecticides, organophosphates, carbamates, and nerve agents.	Remember **SLUDGE**: **S**aliva, **L**acrimation, **U**rination, **D**efecation, **G**I upset, and **E**mesis. Early on tachycardia; lethargic; paralysis; shock; anxiety; bronchospasms; ataxia; pulmonary edema; bradypnea; seizure; and coma. Bradycardia in late stages.	Wash toxins off the patient. If oral ingestion within 1 hour, give 1 g/kg charcoal. Atropine may reverse central nervous system effects. Ipratropium bromide (Atrovent)–nebulized treatment may dry secretions. Administer pralidoxime or obidoxime as ordered. Pralidoxime should *not* be administered without concurrent atropine.
Alcohol abuse Liquors, beers, wines, moonshine, rubbing alcohol, even mouthwash. Vaping or use of alcohol-soaked tampons are also methods of ingesting alcohol.	Slurred speech; unsteady gait; hypoglycemia, and alcohol odor. The patient may go into withdrawal.	Obtain alcohol level. IV banana bag and time for alcohol levels to drop. Glucose benzodiazepines such as lorazepam (Ativan) are used to treat and prevent further progression of withdrawal.
Anticholinergic overdose Antihistamines, antidepressants, dicyclomine, tropicamide, alkaloids cyclopentolate, homatropine, phenothiazines, amanita muscaria, jimsonweed or deadly nightshade, belladonna, atropine, and tricyclics.	Mnemonic: Blind as a bat, mad as a hatter, red as a beet, hot as hare, dry as a bone, the bowel and bladder lose their tone, and the heart runs along. Respectively, pupillary dilation—blurred vision; delusions, hallucinations, or delirium; hyperthermia; dry mucosa and skin; GI and bladder paralysis; and tachycardia. Cardiovascular collapse; seizure; hypertension; thirst.	Charcoal 1 g/kg within 1 hour of ingestion. Supportive measures, benzodiazepines for agitation and seizures. Antidote: Physostigmine in cases with both peripheral and central signs of anticholinergic poisoning and 1 g/kg charcoal if ingestion was less than 1 hour ago.

Anticoagulants—oral Direct thrombin inhibitor Dabigatran (Pradaxa)	Bleeding.	Antidote: Idarucizumab (Praxbind)—Life-threatening bleeding or emergent/invasive procedure. IV 5 g (administered as 2 separate 2.5-g doses no more than 15 minutes apart). Hemodialysis.
Factor Xa inhibitor Rivaroxaban (Xarelto) Apixaban (Eliquis) Edoxaban (Savaysa) Betrixaban (Bevyxxa)	Bleeding	Antidote: Andexanet alfa (Andexxa) Only for severe life-threatening bleeding (e.g., intracranial hemorrhage) off-label use for edoxaban and betrixaban. Kcentra (PCC) IV 2,000 units × 1 or 25–50 units/kg × 1.
Warfarin (Coumadin, Jantoven)	Bleeding.	Obtain prothrombin time and INR level, and give phytonadione (vitamin K) onset of action: PO 6–10 hours; IV 1–2 hours. PCC for acute major bleeding or urgent surgery/invasive procedure. Onset of action; within 10 minutes.
Anticoagulants—parenteral LMWH Enoxaparin (Lovenox)	Bleeding.	Antidote: Protamine partial reversal agent
Heparin	Bleeding.	Obtain partial thromboplastin time level and antidote: protamine sulfate

(continued)

Table 22.1

Substance Abuse and Toxicology Table (*continued*)

Drug/Substance	Signs and Symptoms	Interventions/Anticipated Orders
Benzodiazepines Depressants and sedatives such as Valium, Serax, Xanax, Ativan, Klonopin, Versed, and Rohypnol aka "roofies" which are 10 times as potent as diazepam.	Drowsiness; amnesia; confusion; bradypnea; cool clammy skin; dilated pupils; sedation; and hypotension.	Support measures fluids and/or vasopressors for hypotension. Respiratory depression/failure intubation. Antidote: Flumazenil (Romazicon) Only utilize in acute life-threatening ingestion. Do NOT use in patients who are chronically on benzodiazepines. Reversal ma cause life-threatening seizures and withdrawal.
Beta-blockers Atenolol, metoprolol, propranolol, and sotalol.	Bradycardia; hypotension; shock; and cardiac arrest.	Hypotension: fluids and vasopressors. Glucagon 3–10 mg IV bolus. IV Calcium Chloride or gluconate. Hyperinsulinemia-euglycemia therapy. Atropine for symptomatic bradycardia and prepare pacemaker
Caffeine Powder/Capsules Concentrated OTC caffeine. 2 tsp= **(10,000 mg)** lethal dose (like drinking 70 Red Bulls at one time)	Tachycardia, seizures, hypertension, dysrhythmias, coma, and death in high doses.	If recent ingestion charcoal may be helpful. IV fluids, EKG, Beta-blockers (esmolol), procainamide, lidocaine, bicarbonate. Vasopressin or phenylephrine if hypotension occurs. Dialysis or intralipid therapy may be helpful.
Calcium channel blockers Verapamil, nifedipine (Procardia), and diltiazem.	Bradycardia; hypotension; lethargy; confusion; bradypnea; nausea and vomiting; shock; hyperglycemia; and cardiac arrest.	Calcium Chloride 10–20 mg/kg (max 2 g) or calcium gluconate 60 mg/kg (max 3–6 g) intravenously over 5 minutes until response seen. Significant hypercalcemia may be necessary before severely intoxicated patients respond. Give normal saline bolus and vasopressors for hypotension. Hyperinsulinemia-euglycemia therapy

Carbon monoxide poisoning Carbon monoxide displaces oxygen on the hemoglobin.	Hypoxia; confusion; headache; nausea and vomiting; dizziness; coma; seizures; cyanosis; and death.	Give oxygen via nonrebreather mask; provide hyperbaric oxygen treatment; and obtain carbon dioxide levels.
Cardiac glycosides Digoxin, digitoxin, oleander, and foxglove.	Visual yellow-green halos; nausea and vomiting; headache; bradycardia; hyper- and hypokalemia, ventricular arrhythmias; shock; and cardiac arrest.	Obtain digoxin level; charcoal 1 g/kg within 1 hour of ingestion. Give digoxin (Digibind) immune fab dose dependent on digoxin dose ingested; 1 mg/kg lidocaine intravenously for arrhythmias, and atropine for bradycardia.
DXM Cough suppressant found in over-the-counter cold medications. Street names: triple C; CCC; dexing; skittles, velvet; poor man's PCP; rojo; and robo tripping.	Confusion; hallucinations; lethargy; slurred speech; hypertension; eye spasms; paranoia; tachycardia; vomiting; seizures; coma, and death.	Many cold medications have other medications such as acetaminophen, pseudoephedrine, and guaifenesin to consider. Treatment is supportive. Antidotes and screening for DXM is currently unavailable.
Ethylene glycol (antifreeze)	First 1–12 hours: Slurred speech; inebriated; coma; seizure; and death. 12–24 hours: tachycardia; hypertension; tachypnea; congestive heart failure; acute respiratory distress syndrome; and cardiac collapse. 24–72 hours: nephrotoxicity; flank pain; renal failure; and hypocalcemia.	Labs: Determine serum ethylene glycol level; prepare basic metabolic panel; and obtain urinalysis. Give gastric lavage (charcoal is ineffective). Antidote: Give fomepizole therapy immediately; seizure control: benzodiazepines, hypocalcemia-induced seizures 10% 10–20 mL calcium gluconate intravenously. Metabolic acidosis 50 mEq IV sodium bicarbonate; cofactor therapy: pyridoxine IV 100 mg; 2 g IV magnesium; 100 mg IV thiamine; 15 mg/kg IV fomepizole (Antizol); and prepare for dialysis.

(continued)

Table 22.1

Substance Abuse and Toxicology Table (*continued*)

Drug/Substance	Signs and Symptoms	Interventions/Anticipated Orders
GHB acid Depressant sold as liquid or dissolvable white powder. Street names: Easy Lay, G, Georgia Home Boy, Goop, Grievous Bodily Harm, Liquid Ecstasy, Liquid X, and Scoop.	Low doses produce euphoria, lethargy, reduced anxiety, confusion, and memory loss. High doses produce bradycardia, bradypnea, hypothermia, nausea, vomiting, seizures, unconsciousness, coma, and death.	Support ABCs and treat the symptoms. No toxicologic screening or current antidote exists. GHB analogues can cause liver and kidney damage; check liver function tests and metabolic panel. Supportive therapy; withdrawal symptoms: tachycardia, anxiety, tremors, hypertension, insomnia, and psychotic thoughts.
Hallucinogens Mushrooms; Ketamine; Ecstasy/MDMA; PCP; LSD abuse and perennial herb Salvia divinorum. Street names: Acid, blotter, Shrooms, Mind Candy, Doses, Fry, Special K, Sally D, and vitamin K.	Agitation; hallucinations; **dilated pupils**; **hyperthermia**; hypertension; bradypnea; seizures; tachycardia; and respiratory arrest.	Reassure and reorient to reality; instruct patient to keep eyes open; and provide good lighting to decrease shadows. Give benzodiazepines for agitation.
Insulin	Weakness; lethargic; syncope; and blood sugar <80.	Monitor blood sugar; give 1-amp dextrose (D50) intravenously, if alert feed the patient a meal; give IM glucagon as ordered if IV access is unobtainable; persistent hypoglycemia may require dextrose continuous infusion (D10).

Iron	Initially: hypotension; nausea; vomiting; and bloody stools. Late (2–3 days): coagulopathies; metabolic acidosis; hemorrhage; renal failure; liver failure; and shock.	Deferoxamine mesylate (Desferal) binds with iron and is excreted via the kidneys.
Marijuana Concentrates 4–6× stronger than top-shelf marijuana. Street names: 710 (oil flipped and backwards) wax, earwax, honeycomb, budder, butane hash oil, BHO shatter, dabs, black glass, and errl, e-cigarettes, and vaporizers make it odorless and smokeless. THC can legally be purchased in some states in the form of gummies and unknowingly overdose.	Paranoia, anxiety, panic attacks, nausea, abdominal pain, cyclic vomiting, hallucinations, psychosis, tachycardia, asthma exacerbation, hypertension. Withdrawal, addiction, and cyclic vomiting problems may occur.	Support ABCs. No antidotes exist, treatment is supportive. Benzodiazepines may help anxiety. IV fluids and antiemetics may be used for nausea and abdominal pain. Haldol may help with cyclic vomiting.
MDMA Colorful pills, powder, or liquid stimulant/psychedelics: Street names: Ecstasy, X, STP, Hug drug; Lover's Speed; Beans; Disco Biscuit, E; Go; Eve; and XTC Ecstasy, Molly.	Euphoria; increased trust; tachycardia; hypertension; **hyperthermia**; sweating; muscle cramps; sexual arousal; chills; confusion; depression; and blurred vision. SIADH.	Treatment is supportive. Treat ABCs first. Cooling blanket or device may be ordered to regulate temperature. Check metabolic panel. Treat any electrolyte imbalances (hyponatremia). Head CT. Consider activated charcoal if recent ingestion.
Nonspecific or unknown	Varies. Complete a thorough assessment and patient history for any clues.	Treat symptoms. Consider activated charcoal in water or 1 g/kg sorbitol.

(continued)

Table 22.1

Substance Abuse and Toxicology Table (*continued*)

Drug/Substance	Signs and Symptoms	Interventions/Anticipated Orders
Narcotics (opioids) Morphine, methadone, dextromethorphan, heroin, (synthetic opioid) meperidine (Demerol), codeine, diphenoxylate, propoxyphene, and synthetic opioids fentanyl (100× more potent than morphine) and carfentanil (10,000× more potent than morphine). Fentanyl and Demerol can be negative in UDS.	**Pinpoint pupils** (miosis), central nervous system depression, depression, bradycardia, flushed face, hypotension, constipation, cool clammy skin, and bradypnea.	Protect airway and provide rescue breaths as needed. IV 0.4–2 mg **naloxone (Narcan)** q2–3min, if no response observed after 10 mg total, consider other causes of respiratory depression. If no IV access can also be IM, IN, or nebulized. Naloxone action is shorter than most opioids **repeat doses or continuous infusion may be required**. Can be obtained over the counter and may have been given on scene. Can lead to agitation and withdrawal symptoms.
Neuroleptics Metoclopramide, haloperidol, thioxanthenes, and phenothiazines.	EKG changes (prolonged QT segments); dysrhythmias; and altered level of consciousness.	Activated charcoal within 1 hour of ingestion. Supportive therapy: extrapyramidal symptoms: Diphenhydramine or benztropine (Cogentin) blocks dopamine reuptake. Neuroleptic malignant syndrome: benzodiazepines; IV crystalloid fluids.
NSAIDs (e.g., ibuprofen, naproxen, ketorolac, meloxicam)	Nausea; vomiting; abdominal pain; drowsiness; tarry or bloody stools; hemoptysis; shallow breathing; syncope; or coma.	Activated charcoal within 1–2 hours post ingestion; supportive care; maintain ABCs; gastric lavage if acute ingestion of massive amounts; hemodialysis to correct acidosis; benzodiazepines for seizures; metabolic acidosis: sodium bicarbonate.

Salicylates Aspirin	Nausea and vomiting; tinnitus; diaphoresis; acidosis; altered mental status; seizures; and shock.	Charcoal within 1 hour of ingestion. However, salicylates are absorbed erratically. Charcoal may be beneficial beyond 1 hour. Fluid resuscitation. Serum and urine alkalization: Sodium bicarbonate bolus 1–2 mEq/kg, then continuous infusion to maintain 1–2 mL urine/kg/hr. Monitor hypokalemia and cautiously replace. Seizure: benzodiazepines; hypoglycemia: dextrose; dialysis for enhanced elimination.
Stimulants (sympathomimetics) Aminophylline, amphetamines, cocaine, ephedrine, caffeine, methylphenidates, methamphetamines, and PCP. Yaba: Meth + Caffein Wasping: Meth + bug spray.	Hypertension; **dilated pupils**; tachycardia; paranoia; vasoconstriction; **hyperthermia**; seizures; chest pain; **acute myocardial infarction**; coma; stoke; (hypotension with caffeine); altered mood; and death.	Activated charcoal within 1 hour of ingestion. Agitation, anxiety, psychosis, and seizure control: benzodiazepines or haloperidol. Hypertension: sedation with benzodiazepines, nitroglycerin, or nitroprusside (Nipride) for hypertension. Avoid beta-blockers.
Synthetic cannabinoids Inhaled synthetic marijuana is commonly marketed as herbal incense or potpourri. Street names: K-2, Spice, Crazy Clown, Blaze, Demon, Black Magic, Ninja, Smoke, Skunk, Yucatan, Fire, and Red X Dawn.	Relaxation; euphoria; anxiety; tachycardia; hypertension; pallor; diaphoresis; delusions; paranoia; psychosis; hallucinations; seizures; nausea and vomiting; loss of consciousness; and aggressive or violent behavior toward self or others. May lead to renal failure.	Antidotes and routine toxicology screening for synthetic cannabinoids are currently unavailable. Treatment is supportive. Benzodiazepines may be ordered for agitation or seizures. Antiemetics may be ordered for nausea. IV fluids may be ordered to correct any electrolyte imbalances.

(continued)

Table 22.1

Substance Abuse and Toxicology Table (*continued*)

Drug/Substance	Signs and Symptoms	Interventions/Anticipated Orders
Synthetic cathinones Oral, inhaled, or injectable synthetic stimulants know as bath salts, alpha-PVP, and Flakka. Street names: Ivory wave, Pure Ivory, Red Dove, Vanilla Sky, White Dove, White Lightning, Cloud Nine, Ocean Burst, and Purple Wave.	Stimulant effects; sweating; palpitations; tachycardia; hallucinations; dilated pupils; paranoid; psychosis; aggressive violent behavior toward self or others; anxiety; agitation; hyperthermia; hypertension can lead to renal failure or myocardial infarction.	Antidotes and routine toxicology screening for synthetic cathinones are currently unavailable. Treatment is supportive. Benzodiazepines can help with agitation and seizures. Restraints may be ordered for safety. Antipsychotics may be given with caution as they tend to lower seizure thresholds.
TCA Amitriptyline, desipramine, nortriptyline, and imipramine.	Tachycardia; nausea; vomiting; tachydysrhythmias; hypotension; seizures; shock; and cardiac arrest.	Activated charcoal within 1 hour of ingestion. Antidote: None. Supportive therapy: Impaired cardiac conduction. Give IV sodium bicarbonate for TCA to obtain serum pH of 7.50–7.55 to alter protein binding; refractory cardiac conduction: hypertonic saline; hypotension: fluid resuscitation and norepinephrine (Levophed). Seizures: benzodiazepines.

Tylenol (acetaminophen) overdose Can lead to liver failure and death. Toxic doses destroy hepatocytes resulting in liver damage and necrosis. 140 mg/kg is toxic. Tylenol can also be mixed or cut in OTC or street drugs such as "cheese" (heroin cut with Tylenol pm).	First 24 hours: asymptomatic; minor GI upset. 24–72 hours: elevated liver function test or renal failure. 72–96 hours: jaundice; renal failure; coagulopathy; and liver necrosis. 4 days to 2 weeks: symptoms resolve or patient dies.	Labs: acetaminophen level 4 hours after ingestion utilize Rumack-Matthew nomogram. Activated charcoal within 1 hour of ingestion. Antidote: Administer NAC (Acetadote Mucomyst, available IV and PO, respectively), the sooner the better; may be useful up to 72 hours after ingestion. Monitor for anaphylactic reactions to NAC which is more common in the IV formulation and asthmatics.
Venom of rattlesnakes, cottonmouth/ water moccasins, and copperheads.	Bite/fang marks with redness/bruising; pain; and swelling.	Antidote: Antivenom, crotalidae polyvalent (CroFab) initial dose 4–6 vials or 8–12 vials in life-threatening effects (shock serious active bleeding). Repeat doses of 4–6 vials if control not achieved. Maximum initial dose: 12 vials. Maintenance dose: 2 vials every 6 hours up to 18 hours. Normal saline for mild symptoms.

ABCs, airway, breathing, and circulation; BHO, butane honey oil; CCC, Coricidin HBP Cough & Cold; DXM, dextromethorphan; GHB, gamma-hydroxybutyric acid; GI, gastrointestinal; IM, intramuscular; IN, intranasal; INR, international normalized ratio; IV, intravenous; LMWH, low-molecular-weight heparin; LSD, D-lysergic acid diethylamide; MDMA, 3,4-methylenedioxy-methamphetamine; NAC, N-acetylcysteine; NSAIDs, nonsteroidal anti-inflammatory drugs; OTC, over-the-counter; PCC, prothrombin complex concentrate; PCP, phencyclidine; PO, by mouth; PVP, pyrrolidinopentiophenone; SIADH, syndrome of inappropriate antidiuretic hormone; STP, Serenity, Tranquility, and Peace; TCA, tricyclic antidepressants; THC, tetrahydrocannabinol; UDS, urine drug screen; XTC, Ecstasy.

SUMMARY

You now have a stronger knowledge base for substance abuse and toxicology emergencies. You should be able to differentiate the types of substance abuse and toxicology emergencies and know how to respond. Because urine drug screens don't screen everything, get an accurate history and complete physical assessment. Check for contents such as pills, bottles, illicit substances, pipes, or any additional information to help identify the causative agent. Tablets/capsules can be identified by using drug references, poison control, or the pharmacy department. Each overdose case is different. Many factors will affect the treatment, including time of ingestion, amount of substance, patient's weight, and current vital signs. Be sure to **contact poison control for every case.** They will help you and the provider come up with the proper individualized treatment course needed.

23

Traumatic Emergencies

Even if you don't work at a trauma center, trauma patients come to all accident and emergency departments. It is important not to become distracted by the obvious traumatic injury such as an amputated limb and adhere to your trauma assessments. Because a trauma patient can hemorrhage to death in just a matter of minutes, you may need to reprioritize your assessment of airway, breathing, and circulation (ABC) to (CAB) circulation, airway, then breathing. This will allow you to **control any external bleeding first,** drastically improving your patient's mortality rate. This chapter will give you a brief overview of some basic trauma situations. It is highly recommended that you sign up for additional advanced trauma training by registering for a local Trauma Nurse Core Course (TNCC) near you.

During this part of your orientation locate and become familiar with

- C-Spine immobilization devices
- Slide or transfer boards
- Rapid infusers
- Vaseline dressing
- Type and Screen, blood bank
- Massive blood transfusion protocol
- Blood warmers, tubing
- Trauma assessment documentation
- Trauma protocol
- Thoracentesis tray
- Chest tubes and drainage systems

- Vented chest seal dressings
- Tourniquets
- Medications to know: dopamine, norepinephrine, dobutamine, milrinone, vasopressin, phenylephrine

TRAUMA PATIENT ASSESSMENT

In real life the trauma team is performing several of these assessment steps simultaneously. However, if you were to take all the assessments and interventions and prioritize in order of most important to least important, you would end up with the assessment below. If your patient is arriving via EMS, you have time to gather equipment, team members, and prepare the room. Once the patient arrives you should perform a quick **across the room assessment**: as you look across the room and see the patient you should be looking for any uncontrolled hemorrhaging, alertness, color, and work of breathing. **If uncontrolled bleeding is noted reprioritize your ABCs to CBA.** The rest of the trauma assessment is as easy as your ABCs, literally. At any time, you notice something is wrong during your assessment, stop and correct and reassess before moving on to the next part of your assessment.

Primary Survey

A. Alertness & Airway-**maintaining C-spine**:
B. Breathing
C. Circulation & Control any hemorrhage
D. Disability (Neurological assessment)
E. Exposure & Environmental control
F. Full Set of Vital Signs & Family Presence
G. Get Monitoring Devices & Give Comfort using the **LMNOP** mnemonic
    l. Laboratory tests
    m. Monitor Cardiac performance
    n. Nasogastric or Orogastric tube insertion
    o. Oxygenation & Ventilation
    p. Pulse oximetry and Pain Management

Notes: ____

Secondary Survey

H. History and Head to Toe Assessment
I. Inspect the Posterior Surfaces
J. Just Keep Reevaluating: the primary survey, vital signs, pain, and any injuries found.

Now that your assessment is complete, you should be able to identify which diagnostic tests and interventions are needed and prepare to admit or transfer the patient.

Notes: ____

TRAUMA TRIAD OF DEATH

If you have ever heard a colleague say, "better to be warm and dead than cold and dead," during a traumatic resuscitation, you colleague is absolutely right. There are three components that will cause your trauma patient to bleed out faster and spiral down quickly to an eminent death, and hypothermia is one of them. See Figure 23.1.

Avoid the Trauma Triad of Death on all your trauma patients by:

- Keeping them warm
- Correcting Acidosis
- Improve clotting formation by transfusing whole blood (platelets, plasma, and Packed Red Blood Cells (PRBCs)

Notes: ____

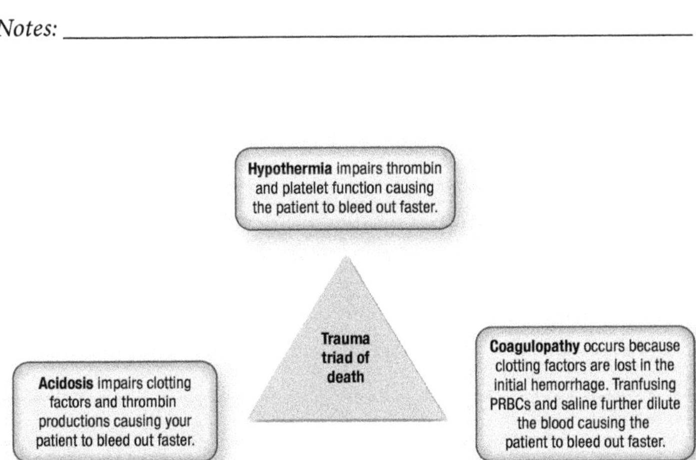

Figure 23.1 Trauma Triad of Death diagram.

Nearly half of trauma patients have ingested some form of alcohol or recreational drugs prior to the traumatic event. Consider **drug and alcohol screenings** on all trauma patients.

ROAD BURN OR ROAD RASH

Road burn/rash is a type of friction *abrasion.*

- *Causes:* Skin friction contact with the "road" or pavement or other abrasive material. It commonly occurs in motorcycle collisions when the patient is not wearing protective gear.
- *Signs and symptoms:* Painful abrasions or large areas of skin that are "rubbed off." Imbedded debris or asphalt may be visible.
- *Interventions:* Treat any life-threatening injuries first. Road rash is very painful; anticipate orders to apply local or topical anesthetics or administer pain medication prior to wound cleansing with vigorous scrubbing. Once the local or topical anesthesia has had the desired effect, you will need to cleanse the wound, removing any debris. Personally, I like to use those surgical chlorhexidine scrub sponges with a sponge on one side and a soft brush on the other and normal saline to cleanse the wound. Next, you may anticipate an order to apply antibiotic ointment and a non-adhesive dressing to the wounds.

Notes: ____

____

____

____

____

____

____

____

____

STABBINGS

- *Causes:* Forced penetration by a sharp object, commonly a knife.
- *Signs and symptoms:* Vary depending on the location, bleeding, tissue damage, organ damage, and signs of hypovolemic shock.
- *Interventions:* Note the size, length, and type of weapon used and location of injury; control bleeding with pressure and/or hemostatic dressing; monitor cardiac rhythm and blood pressure. Contact local law enforcement according to state law and hospital policy. Place any removed clothing in a paper bag and maintain chain of custody for forensic evidence. Anticipate orders to start two large-bore IVs; obtain type and crossmatch for blood transfusion; give emergency blood transfusion, as ordered, if patient is in hypovolemic shock; and anticipate possible operating room (OR) admission.

Notes: ____

____

____

____

____

____

____

____

____

____

____

____

____

____

____

THORACIC TRAUMAS

These traumas may be the result of motor vehicle collisions, gunshot wounds, falls, blasts, blows to the chest, or crushing injuries.

Pneumothorax: An air leak in the pleural space resulting in partial or total collapse of the lung.

- *Causes:* A traumatic lung injury or spontaneous rupture that results in an air leak into the pleural space.
- *Signs and symptoms:* Sucking chest wound; dyspnea; tachypnea; tachycardia; sudden pleuritic chest pain; anxiety; restlessness; diminished or absent breath sounds on affected side; pallor; hypotension if severe; subcutaneous emphysema; palpitations; or asymptomatic if small.
- *Interventions:* Put patient in high Fowler's position; give oxygen; cover open chest wounds with flap Vaseline gauze dressing secured on three sides or a vented chest seal; anticipate orders to check pulse oximetry, connect to cardiac monitor, arrange for immediate chest x-ray, prepare to assist with needle or finger thoracostomy or chest tube insertion, administer pain meds, and obtain Intravenous (IV) access.

Notes: ____

Essential Facts

- Treatment for a sucking chest wound is a three-sided nonporous dressing. However, if the patient's respiratory status deteriorates after application of the three-sided dressing, and signs of a tension pneumothorax (hypotension, distended neck veins, and tracheal deviation) are developing, try **removing** the three-sided dressing. Then reassess the respiratory status.
- Patients on the ventilator with a small pneumothorax can easily develop a tension pneumothorax due to the positive pressure

Hemothorax: Blood leak in the pleural space resulting in partial or total collapse of the lung.

- *Causes:* Penetrating chest trauma with bleeding into the lung.
- *Signs and symptoms:* Blood loss greater than 1,500 mL is considered a massive hemothorax: mediastinal shift (systolic blood

pressure of less than 80 mmHg, and capillary refill of more than 4 seconds); decreased urine output; respiratory distress; hypotension; tachycardia; cyanosis; tracheal deviation; decreased or absent breath sounds; and flat neck veins due to hypovolemic shock.

- *Interventions:* Treat ABCs; assist with chest tube insertion; anticipate orders to prepare for emergency thoracotomy, open two large-bore IV accesses, administer IV fluid bolus, monitor cardiac performance, and prepare for emergency blood transfusion. If large volume of blood loss, anticipate blood or autotransfusion.

Notes: ____

Essential Facts

Never clamp a chest tube not even for transportation. Doing so can cause a tension pneumothorax!

Flail chest: Fracture of two or more ribs in two or more places resulting in a free-floating segment of the chest wall. Mortality increases if bilateral injury is present.

- *Causes:* Chest trauma.
- *Signs and symptoms:* Paradoxical chest movement; chest pain; dyspnea; tachypnea; and crepitus.
- *Interventions:* Treat ABCs; anticipate orders to start IV access, monitor pulse oximetry, control pain, and prepare for possible intubation for ventilation assistance.

Question: What is the most serious injury associated with fractures of first and second ribs?
Answer: *Aortic rupture.*

Notes: ____

____

____

____

RUPTURED DIAPHRAGM

This is a tear or rupture of the diaphragm; it can be a life-threatening injury.

- *Causes:* Blunt or penetrating forces resulting in herniation of abdominal contents into the thoracic cavity.
- *Signs and symptoms:* Epigastric pain; chest pain; abdominal pain; bowel sounds in lower chest; dyspnea; dysphagia; and decreased breath sounds.
- *Interventions:* Anticipate orders to monitor cardiac performance and pulse oximetry, use nasogastric tube for stomach decompression, establish IV access, and prepare for surgery.

Notes: ____

____

____

____

____

____

____

____

____

____

____

____

____

____

____

SPINAL CORD TRAUMAS

These traumas may result in spinal shock or neurogenic shock.

- *Causes:* Neck or back trauma.
- *Signs and symptoms:* Breathing difficulty; varying paralysis depending on injury location; **bradycardia**; hypotension; autonomic dysreflexia (hypertensive condition: headache, sweating, and bradycardia); warm and dry skin; may assume room temperature (poikilothermia); pain; **loss of voluntary bowel or bladder control,** and possible **priapism.**
- *Interventions:* Open airway maintaining cervical (C-spine) immobilization (use jaw thrust maneuver); conduct a neurological assessment; **use 6-man lift (No Logrolling)**; prepare for possible endotracheal intubation; assist if ventilation assistance required; anticipate orders to administer IV fluids and steroids, insert naso or oragastricoragastric tube and Foley catheter, provide therapeutic hypothermia per hospital policy, and take measures to avoid skin breakdown.

Essential Facts

Assume an existing spinal injury on any trauma patient that has an altered level of consciousness or is intoxicated until proven otherwise. **Maintain spinal immobilization until cleared with radiological studies.**

Question: Children younger than 8 years of age are most likely to have what type of spinal cord injury?
Answer: *Cervical spine C1 to C3*

Notes: ____

____

____

____

____

ABDOMINAL TRAUMAS

Splenic injuries: Trauma or injury to the spleen.

- *Causes:* Usually occurs with blunt left upper quadrant abdominal trauma.
- *Signs and symptoms:* **Kehr's sign** (see Figure 23.2; left upper quadrant abdominal pain that may radiate to the left shoulder); absent or hypoactive bowel sounds; abdominal muscle rigidity; and hypovolemic shock.
- *Interventions:* Frequent abdominal assessments (look, listen, and feel); anticipate orders to establish large-bore IV access; perform focused assessment with sonography in trauma (FAST) ultrasound exam; administer IV fluids, hemoglobin and hematocrit; type and screen blood; and prepare for blood transfusion and surgical intervention. Narrowing pulse pressure may indicate ongoing blood loss.

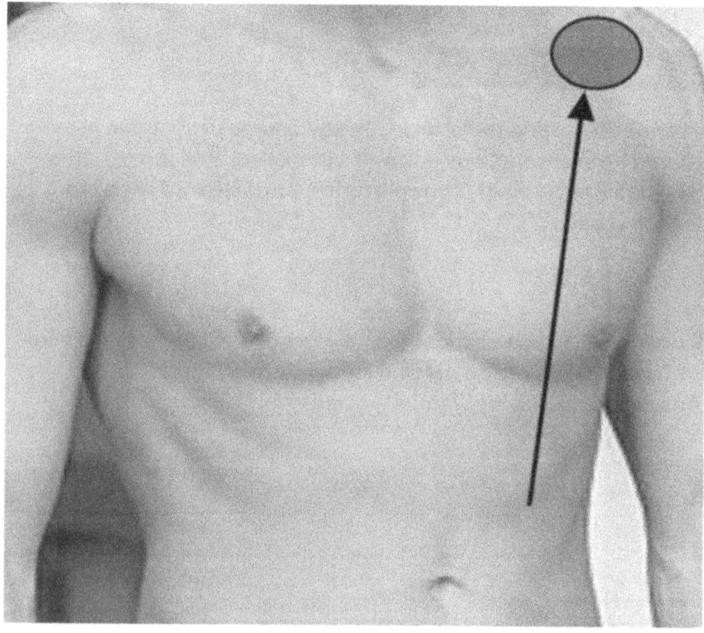

Figure 23.2 Kehr's sign.
Source: Steve Han.

Question: In blunt abdominal trauma, which organs are most commonly injured?
Answer: *The spleen, liver, and bowels.*

Question: Why are injuries to hollow organs difficult to identify?
Answer: *They can leak slowly delaying obvious symptoms for hours or days.*

The highly vascular ruptured spleen is a life-threatening injury. Check Kehr's sign (see Figure 23.2), which is a sharp pain in the left upper abdominal quadrant radiating to the left scapula.

Notes: ____

Pelvic fractures: Either stable or unstable. With a pelvic fracture, your patient can lose up to about 3,000 mL of blood!

- *Causes:* Pelvic trauma.
- *Signs and symptoms:* Pain; pelvic instability; rigidity; hypoactive bowel sounds; hypovolemic shock; and leg shortening or rotation. If urethral laceration: blood from urethral meatus. If bladder laceration: suprapubic pain and an inability to void.
- *Interventions:* Anticipate orders to apply pelvic binder using a **6-man lift, no logrolling**, establish large-bore IV access, administer IV isotonic fluid bolus, arrange for pelvic x-ray or CT scan, type and screen blood, and prepare for possible surgery or interventional radiology.

Notes: ____

Essential Facts

- Logging rolling a patient with a pelvic fracture can lead to fatal hemorrhage. Obtain x-rays or CTs prior to moving the patient or applying a pelvic binder.

Question: What is contraindicated if blood is noted at the urethral meatus?
Answer: *Foley catheter.*

HEAD TRAUMAS

Linear skull fracture: A nondepressed skull fracture.

- *Causes:* Head trauma.
- *Signs and symptoms:* Pain over fracture; scalp laceration; headache; and possible decreased level of consciousness.
- *Interventions:* Elevate head of bed, obtain neurological assessment; clean and dress any wounds; arrange for skull x-rays or head CT scans; and inform patient of head-injury-patient teaching instructions upon discharge.

Notes: ____

Basilar skull fracture: A fracture to the bones at the base of the skull. Complications include infection and cerebrospinal fluid (CSF) leak.

- *Causes:* Head trauma to base of skull.
- *Signs and symptoms:* Altered level of consciousness; bruising behind the ear (**Battle's sign**) 12 to 24 hours after injury; bruising around the eyes (**Racoon's eyes**) 12 to 24 hours after injury; headache; rhinorrhea; otorrhea; and unilateral hearing loss (see Figure 23.3).
- *Interventions:* If there is a CSF leak, apply dry sterile loose dressing below the drainage. Elevate the head of the bed, obtain frequent neurological assessments; anticipate orders to arrange for x-rays and head CT scan, establish IV access, administer antibiotics, and avoid nasogastric tube.

Notes: ____

Depressed skull fracture: A concave-like skull fracture. May be an open fracture; assess for CSF and bleeding.

- *Causes:* Direct blow to the head; head trauma.
- *Signs and symptoms:* Altered level of consciousness; head laceration; headache; and skull depression noted upon palpation.
- *Interventions:* Apply loose sterile dressing; perform frequent neurological assessments; anticipate orders to: establish IV access; administer antibiotics; arrange for operating room admission, x-rays, and head CT scan.

Notes: ____

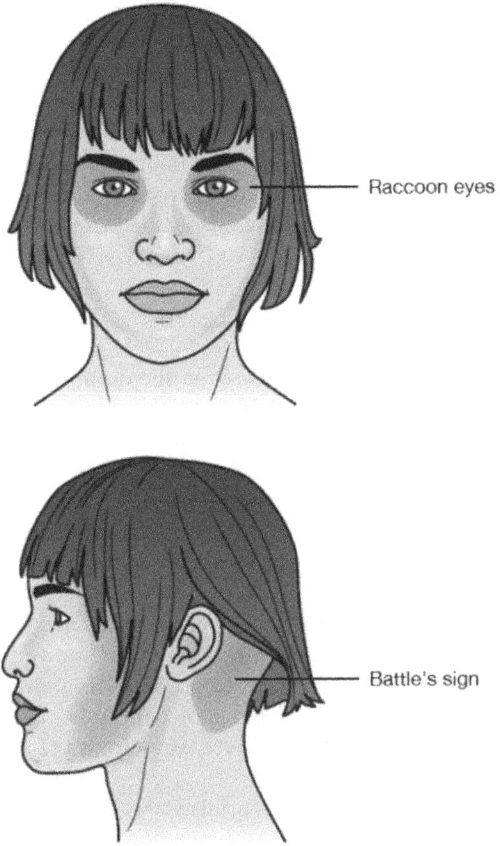

Figure 23.3 Raccoon eyes and Battle's sign.

Essential Facts

A loose sterile dressing is used on a depressed skull fracture and nasally for rhinorrhea to check for CSF leaks.

Concussion or mild diffuse traumatic brain injury: A closed head injury resulting in transient neurological changes with a Glasgow Coma Scale (GCS) of 13 to 15.

- *Causes:* Blunt head or neck trauma.
- *Signs and symptoms:* Nausea; vomiting; dizziness; fatigue; headache; phonophobia; brief altered level of consciousness;

anxiety; irritability; photophobia; poor concentration; normal head CT report; and possible amnesia.

- *Interventions:* Perform a neurological assessment; elevate head of bed; anticipate orders for head CT scan and hospital admission if loss of consciousness lasts more than 5 minutes or patient remains confused, and provide head injury discharge instructions. To promote healing and avoid post-concussive or second impact syndromes, sports activities should be restricted until cleared by provider.

Notes: ____

Subdural hematoma: Bleeding between the dura mater (outermost brain covering) and the arachnoid layer (fine fibrous layer between dura and pia mater) of the meninges resulting in direct pressure on brain tissue surface.

- *Causes:* Commonly caused by head trauma, acceleration and/or deceleration forces, or violent shaking resulting in a tear to the bridging veins.
- *Signs and symptoms:* headache, nausea, vomiting, changes in level of consciousness; deteriorating mental status; fixed and dilated pupil on side of injury; increased intracranial pressure; immediate and prolonged coma; and posturing (de**cort**icate, toward the **cor**d; decerebrate, away from the cord; see Figure 23.4).
- *Interventions:* Perform neurological assessment; anticipate orders for a head CT scan, take measures to reduce intracranial pressure, and prepare patient for neurosurgery.

Notes: ____

Epidural hematoma: Bleeding between skull and dura mater.

- *Causes:* Head trauma. This condition commonly occurs with temporal and parietal skull fractures.
- *Signs and symptoms:* Transient loss of consciousness; ipsilateral pupil dilation; posturing; and hemiparesis.
- *Interventions:* Perform neurological assessment; anticipate orders for a head CT scan, take measures to reduce intracranial pressure, and prepare patient for surgery.

Notes: ____

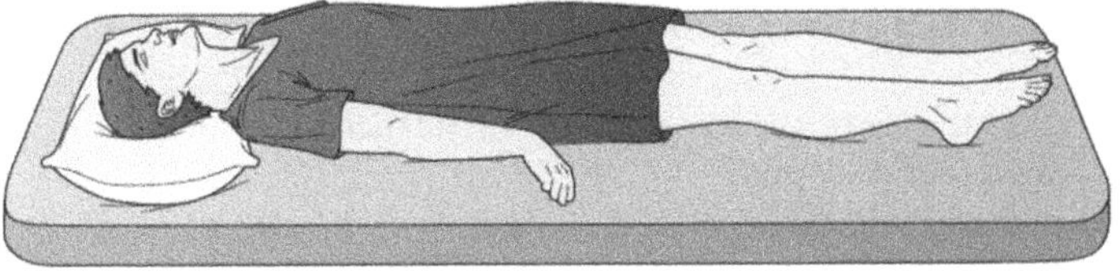

Decerebrate posturing

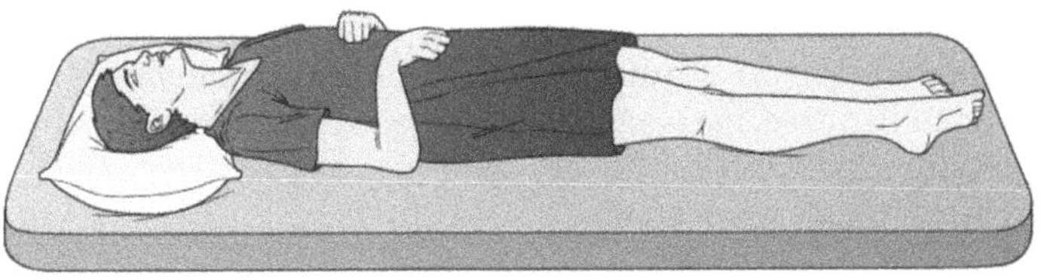

Decorticate posturing

Figure 23.4 Decerebrate and decorticate posturing.

Subarachnoid hemorrhage: Bleeding between pia mater (delicate surface layer of brain) and arachnoid membrane.

- *Causes:* Head trauma. This injury is frequently associated with child abuse and has a high mortality rate.
- *Signs and symptoms:* Headache; nausea and vomiting; altered level of consciousness; neurological deficits; seizure; and posturing.
- *Interventions:* Prepare neurological assessment; anticipate order to arrange for head CT scan; and prepare for surgery.

Notes: ____

Contusion: Bruise to the brain surface.

- *Causes:* Direct blow to the head.
- *Signs and symptoms:* Neurological deficits; altered level of consciousness for more than 6 hours; nausea and vomiting; amnesia; seizure; visual disturbances; and posturing.
- *Interventions:* Perform neurological assessment, immobilize C-spine, arrange for head CT scan when ordered, and provide head-injury-patient teaching upon discharge.

Notes: ____

INCREASED INTRACRANIAL PRESSURE

- *Causes:* Head trauma, electrolyte imbalances, and meningitis.
- *Signs and symptoms:*
  - Early: Altered level of consciousness; headache; nausea/vomiting;
  - Late: Nonreactive, dilated pupils; unresponsiveness; posturing; bradypnea or Cheyne–Stokes respirations; bradycardia; widening pulse pressure; and bulging fontanels in children younger than 2 years of age.
- *Interventions:* Anticipate orders to administer mannitol, administer sedatives, maintain intracranial pressure less than 15 mmHg, elevate head of bed to 30°, avoid hypotension, and avoid Valsalva maneuver.

Notes: ____

SUMMARY

You now have a stronger knowledge base for Traumatic Emergencies. Major trauma emergencies are always critical situations. You should be able to differentiate among the various types of basic trauma and know how to respond. Remember to **control any hemorrhaging as it is one of the most preventable causes of death in a trauma patient.** Complete your trauma assessment and avoid the trauma triad of death. Finding time to chart during a critical emergency is difficult. Most of the time, you need another nurse to help. All A&E nurses have to be team players. Notify your team and volunteer or ask someone to document as care is provided. Rapid responses save lives. To ease any anxiety, take some deep and cleansing breaths, get help, and sign up for a TNCC near you. After a trauma it is good to debrief with the team; talk about what went well and any areas of opportunity.

24

Triage

Although most A&Es have a triage area, **triage is not actually a place but a process**. If you think about it, you can triage a patient anywhere, even in the parking lot! By definition, triage is a French-derived word that means "to choose or to sort." Sorting sounds simple enough. So what is the big deal? Well, the decisions made by the triage nurse determine the level of care and urgency in which a patient will be seen. For instance, say you triage a 21-year-old female with severe right-sided abdominal pain as a level 3 or nonurgent. You think to yourself, "She is not that sick because she looks fine." She waits several hours while all the level 2 or urgent patients are seen by the doctor. When the doctor finally sees her, she is now hypotensive and bleeding internally because her ectopic pregnancy has ruptured. As you can see, the decisions made in triage can directly affect patient outcomes. It sounds scary, but with the right training, experience, and critical thinking skills, you too can master the art of triage. This chapter provides you with some of the tools you will need. After studying this chapter, you should be able to identify which patients can wait and which patients cannot wait, differentiate the levels of triage acuity, perform an across-the-room assessment, and list the common pitfalls of triage.

During this part of your orientation, locate and become familiar with:

- Your facility's triage acuity system and documentation requirements
- Your A&E's triage protocol orders
- Pediatric vital signs

- Your facility's policy on isolation and infection control
- Triage and travel screening process
- Emergency Medical Treatment and Active Labor Act (EMTALA)
- Consent for Minors State Regulations
- Security notification and panic buttons
- The patient liaison or representative
- Your facility's lockdown procedure and policy
- Your facility's "left without being seen" policy
- Location of ice packs, dressings, and triage medication supplies

BEFORE YOU CAN TRIAGE

Not just anyone can be a triage nurse. The weight of the decisions made by the triage nurse is heavy. These decisions require sound critical thinking skills, a strong nursing foundation, the ability to multitask, and excellent interpersonal skills. Most A&Es require a triage nurse to have a certain amount of experience, specific certifications, and evidence of having taken a triage class or competency. The Emergency Nurses Association (ENA) recommends that triage be conducted by an RN or nurse practitioner who has at least one year of experience and received formal triage training. Certifications as a board-certified emergency nurse (BCEN) and in pediatric, cardiac, and trauma care are also recommended. Take the initiative to find out what competencies are required and what triage classes are available at your facility and sign up for them.

Notes: ____

____

____

____

____

____

____

____

____

SAFETY FIRST

While triage can occur anywhere, it commonly occurs at the entry points of the A&E. Essentially, as the triage nurse, you are the front line. You must consider the safety of your patients and yourself. Become familiar with your hospital's infection prevention policies regarding triage. Ask the appropriate travel screening question at the designated time of the patient's arrival and document them. If a patient arrives with symptoms of a respiratory or airborne infection, initiate airborne precautions according to hospital policy. Have the patient wear a mask and assign patients to a negative-pressure room where indicated. Failing to do so may result in spreading infections to others and yourself.

Notes: ____

____

____

____

____

____

____

____

____

____

____

____

____

____

____

____

TRIAGE ACUITY SYSTEMS

Believe it or not, there are a variety of triage acuity systems. While your A&E may use a five-level triage acuity system, one of the neighboring A&Es may be using a three-level triage acuity system. The first thing you must do is identify the triage system your A&E is using. Table 24.1 demonstrates some of the differences among the various systems.

Notes: ____

____

____

____

____

____

____

____

____

____

____

Table 24.1

Comparing Triage Systems				
Level	Five-Level Systems	Four-Level Systems	Three-Level Systems	Two-Level Systems
1	Resuscitation	Life threatening	Emergent	Emergent
2	Emergent	Emergent	Urgent	Non-emergent
3	Urgent	Urgent	Nonurgent	
4	Nonurgent	Nonurgent		
5	Referred			

Level 1 or resuscitation: Requires immediate life-saving interventions.
Level 2 or emergent: A high-risk situation, confused/lethargic/disoriented patient, in severe pain or distress, or has dangerously abnormal vital signs.
Level 3 or urgent: Requires many resources.
Level 4 or nonurgent: Requires just one resource.
Level 5 or referred: Requires no resources.

EMERGENCY SEVERITY INDEX

Although there are many different triage systems, the latest research conducted by the ENA supports the use of a five-level system such as the Emergency Severity Index (ESI). See Figure 24.1. Similar five-level triage scales are the Canadian Triage and Acuity Scale, Australasian Triage Scale, and the Manchester Triage System.

Notes: ____

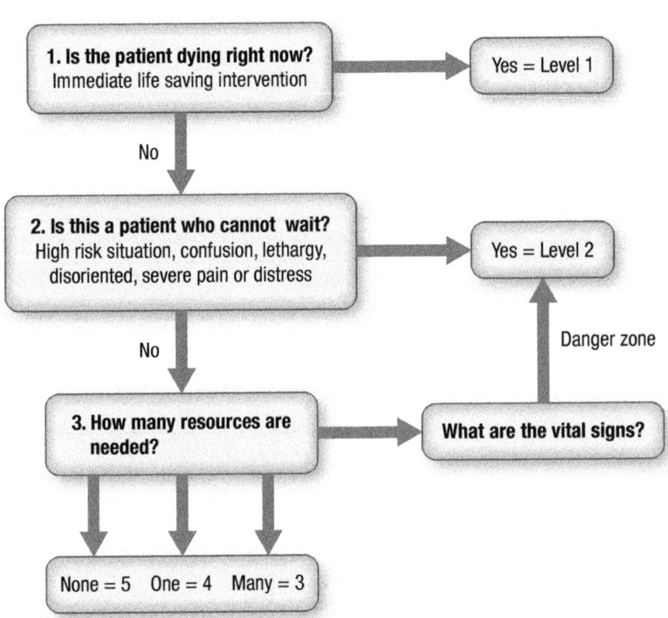

Figure 24.1 Emergency Severity Index level algorithm.

Essential Facts

ESI level is determined by answering four simple questions:

- Is the patient dying or in need of life-saving interventions?
- Is this a patient who will deteriorate if they are placed in the waiting room?
- How many resources are needed?
- What are the vital signs?

RESOURCES

The next question you may be asking is, "What exactly is a resource?" Resources consist of labs, CT, x-ray, MRI, specialty consults, simple procedures, intravenous fluids or medications, intramuscular medications, and inhaled medications. Complex procedures such as moderate sedation count as two resources. However, do not be fooled! There are some interventions that do *not* actually count as a resource. These include simple intravenous access, pelvic exam, point-of-care testing, PO medications, consult to the patient's primary physician, simple dressings, slings, crutches, and splints.

Notes: ____

CHOOSING AN ACUITY LEVEL

Now that you know which triage system your facility is using, you will need specific information to select the appropriate acuity level. First you will need an "across-the-room" assessment, followed by a chief complaint, interview with patient, vital signs, and focused physical exam.

- *Across-the-room assessment:* This is exactly as it reads. What do you see when you look across the room as the patient approaches the triage desk? In order to do this well, the triage nurse must be in a position to view the entire waiting room. Things to look for include the following:
  - *General appearance:* Alert or unresponsive, crying, laughing, talking, any obvious deformities, or bloody clothing.
  - *Work of breathing:* Labored or unlabored, coughing, drooling, gasping, wheezing, rapid or slow respiratory rate, or use of accessory muscles.
  - *Circulation:* Pink or pale, diaphoretic, flushed, normal, or jaundice.

If you find an unstable patient entering the waiting room, do not delay care. If they are unstable, bypass the triage area altogether and take the patient to a bed to begin treatment. For example: If a family member wheels a pale, diaphoretic, unresponsive patient into the waiting room, do *not* stop to take vital signs and interview the patient! The patient is unresponsive. Bring the patient back for treatment immediately. Remember, triage is a process, not a place; it can be done in the back simultaneously as the patient receives care.

- *Elicit chief complaint:* The first question to ask is, "What brought you in to see us today?" Certain chief complaints can carry higher risks than others. For example, chest pain would be a higher-risk chief complaint than toe injury. The patient with chest pain could be having a fatal heart attack, whereas toe injuries, though painful, are not usually fatal.
- *Interview the patient:* Triage is not the time to conduct an entire head-to-toe assessment. Your goal in triage is to elicit the essential facts needed to make an acuity decision. You should be asking questions that relate to the chief complaint. Look over the triage document at your facility. Most A&E triage screening tools include the following:

- Duration of the chief complaint
- Related symptoms
- Mechanism of injury
- Medical history
- Current medications (prescription or nonprescription)
- Immunizations
- Last menstrual period
- Allergies
- Height and weight
- Department-specific screening questions

- *Obtain vital signs:* Vital signs can influence your final acuity section. If the patient looks fine, has a normal exam, and tells you, "I just feel dizzy," you might not think too much of it. But once you take the patient's blood pressure and it is 289/132, you will think differently. Be sure to memorize the different age-specific normal average vital signs shown in Table 24.2.
- *Conduct a focused physical assessment:* Now that you have collected your subjective data (what the patient says), it is time to document what you see (objective data). If the patient tells you, "I twisted my ankle," take off his socks and shoes and document what the ankle looks like: swollen, obviously deformed, bruised, edematous? Is it tender upon palpation? Are distal pulses present? Is the patient ambulatory?

Notes: ____

Table 24.2

Age-Specific Normal Vital Signs

Age	Newborn	Infant	Toddler	Preschooler	School Age	Adolescent	Adult
Respirations	40–60	30–63	22–37	20–28	18–25	12–20	12–20
Heart rate	90–205	90–180	80–140	65–120	58–115	50–100	60–100
Systolic blood pressure	67–84	72–104	86–106	89–112	97–115	110–131	120

TRIAGE INTERVENTIONS

Triage simply means to sort, but at times you will need to implement some basic interventions. These interventions may include basic life support, cervical immobilization, isolation procedures, some medications (e.g., aspirin for chest pain), EKG (should precede the triage of a chest pain patient), point-of-care blood glucose, and simple wound care (e.g., splinting or ice packs).

Notes: ____

____

____

____

____

____

____

____

____

____

Essential Facts

- The entire triage process should only take about 2 to 5 minutes. Do not be discouraged at first. Speed and efficiency come with time and practice. Learning to multitask will help. For example, you can apply the blood pressure cuff and pulse oximeter to collect vital signs while interviewing the patient.
- Triage documentation is a legal document and should support your acuity decision. Document both subjective and objective data, behaviors, and quotes when applicable. Do *not* document judgments.
- Always accurately weigh pediatric patients; their medications are based on their *current* weight.

PEDIATRICS

Triaging pediatric patients can be quite different than triaging adults. Treat the patient and the family as one unit. Use of the pediatric assessment triangle (PAT) will help you quickly determine which child is the sickest (see Figure 24.2). If all components of PAT are stable, the child is sick based on concerns of caregiver. Disruption in one component of the PAT, means the child is sicker. Disruption in two or more components of the PAT indicates this is the sickest child. Typically, it is best to start with the least invasive assessment and interventions to the most invasive. For example, a rectal temperature may cause the infant to cry interfering with observational assessments. Provide honest answers with kid-friendly words. Be familiar with the normal vital signs for each age group. Obtain actual weights. Remember that fevers without an obvious infection source will require multiple resources. In addition, grunting, stridor, accessory muscle use, sunken or bulging fontanels, or any petechial or purpuric rashes (Figure 24.3), especially with mental status changes, are a pediatric red flag.

Notes: ____

____

____

____

____

____

____

____

____

____

____

____

____

____

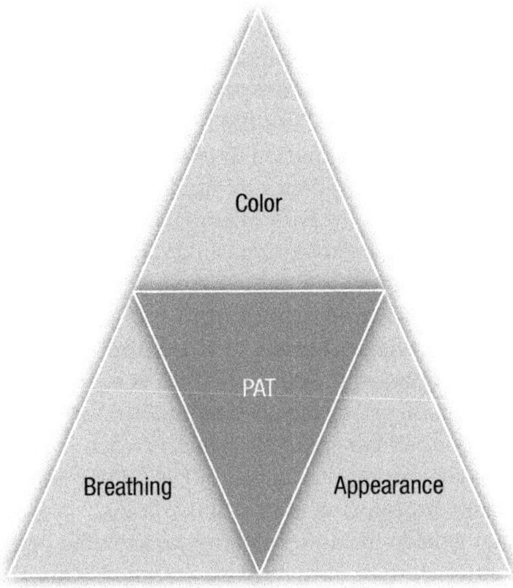

Figure 24.2 Pediatric assessment triangle.

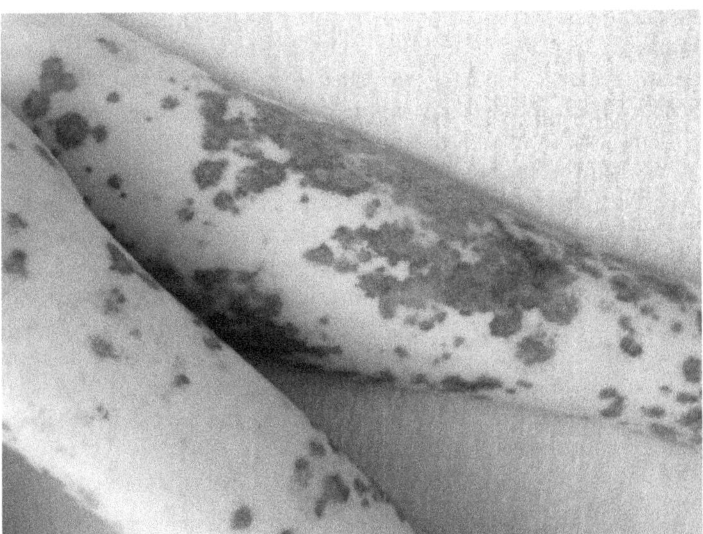

Figure 24.3 Photograph of purpuric rash.
Source: Dr FO. Jr.Tn.

LEGAL ISSUES

If you are the triage nurse, "hospitality" is your middle name! By law, you cannot turn any patient away or even discourage them from seeking emergency medical care. The **EMTALA** is known as the federal "anti-dumping" law. It was enacted in 1986 to prohibit hospitals from refusing to see or transfer financially "undesirable" patients. Prior to this law, patients died in the back of ambulances driving from hospital to hospital, seeking an accepting facility. Under EMTALA, hospitals are obligated to provide a nondiscriminatory medical screening exam to any patient seeking care within 250 yards of the hospital. Understand that a **triage assessment is not typically the same as a medical screening exam unless a provider is at triage**. If a medical emergency condition exists, the hospital is obligated to provide *stabilizing interventions* and *appropriate* transfers when indicated. Failure to uphold this law can result in a fine of $50,000 or more. These laws also apply to any pregnant women in active labor.

Additionally, keep in mind that any person who presents to the hospital seeking medical care must be screened. This also includes minors and those seeking help for mental health or substance abuse. An essential component of being a great triage nurse is knowing your local and state regulations regarding emancipation and care of minor patients, and those individuals with decreased mental capacities. Take the time to look up your state or governing authority's laws regarding legal age for consent. Some exceptions may include emergency medical conditions, emancipated minors, reproductive issues, sexually transmitted infections, drug abuse, or abortion.

Language barriers can cause miscommunications in triage. Be sure to only use hospital-approved translators or language phone service. Document any use of a translator or language phone service. The patient's family members are *not* legal translators, do not allow for patient privacy, and may not translate correctly.

One of your patient's rights is the right to privacy and confidential care. Be sure to interview your patients in as private an area as possible. This may mean pulling the curtain closed or closing the door. Let the patient know you will be asking personal questions and ask if they would like any visitors to leave during the interview. Be aware and monitor the volume of your voice.

Notes: ____

____

____

COMMON PITFALLS OF TRIAGE

Once you spend a little time in triage, you might say to yourself, "Oh, this is not so hard, I've got this." But tread carefully; even the most experienced A&E nurse can be fooled. Following is a list of everyday chief complaints or issues that at first glance appear simple or vague. However, in reality, these might actually be much more emergent than they appear. In triage, you must always assume the worst-case scenario and ask questions to rule out that "worst-case" possibility:

- "I feel weak" or "I am dizzy."
    - *What you might be thinking*: This is a very vague complaint. It could just be the flu, a virus, heat exhaustion, or a fever.
    - *What you should be thinking*: What are the worst things that could make someone feel weak or dizzy? Hypoglycemia, hyperglycemia, dehydration, hypotension or hypertension, hypoxia, sepsis, myocardial infarction, stroke, or arrhythmias.
- "I have a headache."
    - *What you might be thinking*: So do I. The patient just wants pain medication.
    - *What you should be thinking*: What is the worst thing this could be? Hypertension, meningitis, cerebral bleed, brain tumor, head injury, concussion. What is the patient's neurologic status? What is their blood pressure?
- The patient does not look very sick.
    - *What you might be thinking*: If the patient looks fine, it cannot be that bad.
    - *What you should be thinking*: Legally, your opinion does not matter. Look at your subjective and objective data. Is this a high-risk situation?

I once triaged a 73-year-old female having chest pain who "looked fine to me." She was pink, warm, and dry with normal vital signs. She was not clutching her chest, had no previous medical problems, and did not take any medications. She appeared otherwise "healthy." Although I chose the correct acuity level for her, she still surprised me. When we did the EKG, she was having an ST-segment elevated myocardial infarction (STEMI). In layman's terms, she was "having the big one!" She did not display the typical diaphoretic, anxious, and "there is an elephant on my chest" symptoms. Because I chose the correct acuity level, she received timely appropriate care, despite my opinion that she looked fine.

- "I fell."
  - *What you might be thinking*: Treat the injury. If the bleeding is controlled, everything is okay. Ground-level falls are not dangerous.
  - *What you should be thinking*: Why did the patient fall? Hypoglycemia, stroke, hypotension, medication, or arrhythmia. Was the patient dizzy or weak before the fall, or did they trip and fall? Is a head or C-spine injury involved? Is the patient on anticoagulants? Did the patient lose consciousness? What is the neurologic status? Did the patient consume any alcohol or drugs beforehand? Does the patient have a heart condition?
- "My doctor told me to come here."
  - *What you might be thinking*: Those primary care doctors send all their patients here because they do not have time to see them today. If it was serious, they would have called an ambulance or gone to another hospital.
  - *What you should be thinking*: What is the phone number to the primary physician? What tests were performed at the office? What symptoms made the patient call their doctor today? Some patients go to the doctor when they should come to the A&E.
- The patient is not telling you the whole story.
  - *What you might be thinking*: "This does not make any sense." The symptoms do not align with what the patient is saying.
  - *What you should be thinking*: What is the patient's neurologic status? Why does this person think they cannot tell me what is really wrong? Did the patient consume any alcohol or drugs? Do they think you will call the police? Perhaps they think insurance won't pay, or they may be too embarrassed.
- "I feel anxious."
  - *What you might be thinking*: Oh, she has a history of panic attacks; it's just a panic attack. This patient is just being dramatic.
  - *What you should be thinking*: Anxious people get sick too! Has the patient ever felt quite like this before? Hypoxia, anaphylaxis, cardiac event, cerebrovascular accident, even things that are very painful such as bowel obstruction or kidney stones can cause a person to appear "anxious."
- "I have back pain."
  - *What you might be thinking*: Another patient with back pain! They just want pain medication.
  - *What you should be thinking*: Kidney stones, shingles, pyelonephritis, dissecting renal or thoracic aneurysm, or a

spinal injury? Has the patient lost control of their bowels or bladder? Does the pain radiate to the groin or leg? Are there any urinary problems? Is paralysis noted on assessment? Did the pain occur suddenly or gradually?

- "I have been vomiting."
  - *What you might be thinking:* They just need some Zofran and ginger ale and they can go home. It is just another stomach flu.
  - *What you should be thinking*: What is the worst-case scenario of what this could be? Diabetic ketoacidosis, chemotherapy, bowel obstruction, increased intracranial pressure, cardiac problem, food poisoning, or pregnancy. Consider how many times the patient vomited. What is the result of too much vomiting? Electrolyte imbalance and dehydration.
- "My throat is really sore."
  - *What you might be thinking:* It's just strep throat or tonsillitis. I don't really need to look at their tonsils, the doctor will do that. This is a young healthy patient.
  - *What you should be thinking:* What is the worst-case scenario of what this could be? Allergic reaction with swelling to the mouth and airway, toxic ingestion, epiglottitis, or peritonsillar abscess.

Notes: ____

____

____

____

____

____

____

____

____

____

____

____

____

SUMMARY

After reading this chapter, hopefully you have gained some of the tools necessary to triage effectively. When used properly, your new triage skills provide communication of care needed across the entire A&E. With practice, your triage skills will improve, and you will easily identify which patients can wait and which patients cannot wait, differentiate the levels of triage acuity, perform an across-the-room assessment, and list the common pitfalls of triage. Be sure to review your facility's triage requirements and policies. Stick to the facts and the triage algorithm; don't let opinions or biases sway your ESI level selection. Just because something is common doesn't mean that it is normal. Although you may not qualify to triage for some time, you may find it helpful to observe the triage operation and process during your orientation and practice with an experienced preceptor.

Appendices

Appendix A
Common A&E Lab Values

Lab	Normal Value	High-Value Causes	Low-Value Causes
Alanine aminotransferase/serum glutamic pyruvic transaminase (ALT/SGPT)	30–65	Liver damage	
Amylase	25–115	Pancreatitis; cholecystitis	
Anion gap	<11	Diabetic ketoacidosis (DKA)	
Aspartate aminotransferase/ serum glutamic-oxaloacetic transaminase (AST/SGOT)	15–37	Liver damage	Insulin overdose
Beta-hydroxybutyrate	<0.4	Diabetic ketoacidosis	
Blood urea nitrogen (BUN)	7–18	Renal disease	

(continued)

Lab	Normal Value	High-Value Causes	Low-Value Causes
Brain-type natriuretic peptide (BNP) and NT proBNP	Varies by gender and age BNP <100 NT proBNP <300	Right-sided heart failure; pulmonary hypertension; acute pulmonary embolism; or acute coronary syndromes	
Calcium (Ca)	8.5–10.6	Hyperthyroidism; tuberculosis; too much vitamin D	Pancreatitis; parathyroid trauma; alcohol abuse; renal failure
Carboxyhemoglobin level	<1.5%	Carbon monoxide poisoning	
Creatine kinase-MB (CKMB)	0–3.6	Myocardial infarction	
Creatinine	0.6–1.3	Renal disease	
D-dimer	0–682	Congestive heart failure; pulmonary embolism	
Hematocrit (HCT)	37–47	Dehydration	Anemia; gastrointestinal bleeding
Hemoglobin (HGB)	12–16	Dehydration	Anemia; gastrointestinal bleeding
Lactic acid	4.5–19.8	Oxygen deprivation and sepsis	
Lipase	114–286	Pancreatitis; cholecystitis	

(*continued*)

Lab	Normal Value	High-Value Causes	Low-Value Causes
Partial thromboplastin time (PTT)	18–41 (varies)	Hemophilia; heparin overdose; disseminated intravascular coagulation (DIC)	
Platelets (PLT)	140–440	Chronic inflammation	Thrombocytopenia
Potassium (K) CO_2	3.5–5.1 21–32	Metabolic acidosis; respiratory acidosis	Poor potassium intake; diuretics; nausea, vomiting, and diarrhea
Procalcitonin (PCT)	<0.15	Systemic bacterial infection; sepsis	
Prothrombin time (PT)	11–14 (varies)	Coumadin overdose; decreased potassium; liver disease	
Red blood cell (RBC) count	4.2–5.5	Dehydration	Anemia
Sodium (Na)	135–145	Sweating; diarrhea; diabetes	Congestive heart failure; cirrhosis; renal failure; nausea, vomiting, and diarrhea; excess water intake
Troponin	0–0.10	Myocardial infarction	
White blood cell count (WBC)	4–11	Infection; inflammation; leukemia—very high levels	Neutropenia

Appendix B
Everyday A&E Medications

Medication	Dose	Use
Acetaminophen (Tylenol, Datril)	Adult: 650–1,000 mg Max dose: 3,000–4,000 mg/d Children: 10–15 mg/kg; do *not* exceed five doses in 24 hours; max dose 75 mg/kg/d Not to exceed 3,000–4,000 mg/d	Fever and analgesic
Acetaminophen with codeine (Tylenol with codeine)	Doses vary Codeine component of 15– 60 mg. Q4h PO as needed for pain Children: Codeine 0.5–1 mg/kg/dose q4–6h PO as needed for pain; max dose = 60 mg Refer to acetaminophen dosing section.	Opioid analgesic Suspension: acetaminophen 120 mg and codeine 12 mg/5 mL

(continued)

Medication	Dose	Use
Acetylcysteine (Acetadote, Mucomyst)	Adult/children: Oral 72-hour regimen: Loading dose: 140 mg/kg × 1 Maintenance dose: 70 mg/kg q4h× 17 doses; repeat dose if emesis occurs within 1 hour of administration. Acetadote IV 21-hour regimen: Loading dose: 150 mg/kg (max: 15 g) infused over 1 hour Second dose: 50 mg/kg (max: 5 g) infused over 4 hours Third dose: 100 mg/kg (max: 10 g) infused over 16 hours	Antidote for acetaminophen (Tylenol) overdose
Acetylsalicylic acid (aspirin)	75–325 mg PO or by rectum; indication determines dosing interval	Antiplatelet, analgesic, NSAID
Adenosine (Adenocard)	Initial 6 mg rapid IV push over 1–2 seconds. Follow with 20 mL normal saline bolus. Second dose of 12 mg rapid IV push. Children <50 kg: initial 0.05–0.1 mg/kg rapid IV push dose. Second dose 0.1–0.2 mg/kg. Children ≥50 kg refer to adult dosing.	Narrow complex PSVT or SVT; *Not for A-fib, A-flutter, or VT*
Albuterol (Proventil, Ventolin, Proair)	Children: Metered dose inhaler (MDI) 90 mcg/puff; four to eight puffs q20min for three doses, then q1–4h as needed; nebulizer: 0.1–0.15 mg/kg/dose q20min for three doses, then 0.15–3 mg/kg (max: 10 mg) q1–4h as needed. Adult: MDI; four to eight puffs q20min for up to 4 hours, then q1–4h as needed; nebulizer: 2.5–5 mg q20min for three doses, then 2.5–10 mg q1–4h or 10–15 mg/hr continuous.	Bronchodilator for asthma/chronic obstructive pulmonary disease. Also treat hyperkalemia

(continued)

Medication	Dose	Use
Alteplase (Activase)	Wt based dosing refer to hospital protocol for bolus and infusion doses.	Thrombolytic (clot buster); acute ischemic stroke, massive pulmonary embolism, and STEMI
Amiodarone hydrochloride (Cordarone, Nexterone, Pacerone)	150 mg IV over 10 minutes, then 1 mg/min IV for 6 hours, followed by 0.5 mg/min for 18 hours Pulseless VT or VF: 300 mg IV push, second dose 150 mg IV push	Life-threatening ventricular arrhythmias
Atropine sulfate (Atropen)	IV push: 0.5–1 mg q3–5min. Maximum of 3 mg. ET: 2–3 mg in 10 mL normal saline	Symptomatic bradycardia. For organophosphate poisoning, use 2 mg Atropen
Azithromycin (Zithromax)	Adult outpatient pneumonia 500 mg first dose, then 250 mg every day for 4 days. For Chlamydia, 1 g PO for one dose IV: 500 mg/d	Antibiotic commonly used for Chlamydia; PID; and respiratory infections
Banana Bag (1 L D_5 NS or NS, 1 mg folic acid, 10 mL MVI, and 100 mg thiamine) $\pm$ 1–3 g magnesium sulfate	100–250 mL/hr IV	Chronic alcohol abuse and malnourishment
Calcium chloride	200–1,000 mg IV slowly 100 mg/min or 45–90 mg/kg/hr in nonemergent situations. Do *not* mix with sodium bicarbonate or phosphate containing solutions. Central line preferred.	Hyperkalemia, calcium channel or beta-blocker overdose, hypocal-cemia, and magnesium toxicity
Calcium gluconate	One-third potency of calcium chloride 1,000–2,000 mg; do *not* mix with sodium bicarbonate or phosphate-containing solutions; may be administered peripherally.	Hyperkalemia, calcium channel or beta-blocker overdose, hypocal-cemia, and magnesium toxicity

(continued)

Medication	Dose	Use
Ceftriaxone sodium (Rocephin). *For IM can mix with lidocaine 1% as directed on box*	Adult: 250 mg–2 g IV or IM q12–24h. Children: 25–50 mg/kg/ q12h	Antibiotic for infection
Charcoal in water. No sorbitol for a child due to diarrhea/ dehydration.	Infants <1 year: 10–25 g Children 1–12 years: 25–50 g Children >12 years/adults: Initial dose 50–100 g, then 25–50 g q4h	Antidote for toxins. Can mix with chocolate syrup, Coke, or fruit juice for children.
Charcoal with sorbitol	Adult: Refer to charcoal dosing section.	Antidote for toxins
$D_{50}W$, glucose (dextrose)	Average dose 0.5–1 amp intravenous. Check blood sugar.	Acute hypoglycemia; *Use D25 for children.*
Diazepam (Valium). *Do not mix with anything.*	IV: 2–10 mg. Per rectum: 0.2 mg/kg (max: 30 mg)	Seizures and sedation
Digoxin (Lanoxin)	Loading: 0.25–0.6 mg PO or IV	A-fib, A-flutter, heart failure, or SVT
Digoxin immune Fab (Digibind)	Varies depending on digoxin level, with an average 400–800 mg.	Digoxin overdose; digitalis toxicity
Diltiazem hydrochloride (Cardizem)	20 mg (0.25 mg/kg) IV over 2 minutes. May repeat in 15 minutes at 0.35 mg/kg. Continuous infusion: 5–15 mg/hr	A-fib or A-flutter
Dobutamine (Dobutrex)	IV dose: 2.5–40 mcg/kg/min 2.5–20 mcg/kg/min IV for postcardiac arrest	Vasopressor. Pump problems: congestive heart failure without symptoms of shock
Dopamine hydrochloride (Intropin)	IV dose: 5–20 mcg/kg/min. May titrate drip in 5–10 mcg/kg/min increments.	Vasopressor for symptomatic bradycardia, hypotension, or shock

(continued)

Medication	Dose	Use
Enalapril maleate (Vasotec) Enalaprilat (IV formulation)	2.5–40 mg PO daily; IV: 1.25 mg/dose over 5 minutes q6h as needed	Hypertension
Enoxaparin (Lovenox)	0.75–1 mg/kg BID dependent on indication; subcutaneously in abdomen only	Myocardial infarction–anticoagulant
Epinephrine 1:1,000 for subcutaneous/IM administration	SQ or IM (preferred): 0.2–0.5 mg of 1:1,000 solution; may repeat in 20 minutes.	Anaphylaxis and bronchodilator
Epinephrine 1:10,000 IV	IV: 1 mg/10 mL of 1:10,000 solution q3–5min or ET: 2–2.5 mg in 10 mL NS	PEA, asystole, pulseless VT, or VF
Epinephrine IV continuous infusion	Adult: 0.1–0.5 mcg/kg/min titrate to goal BP	Symptomatic bradycardia, or hypotension/shock
Esmolol	Bolus: 500 mcg/kg over 1 minute. Initial dose: 50 mcg/kg/min for 4 minutes. Titrate 50 mcg/kg/min q5min to goal HR/BP. Max: 200 mcg/kg/min	SVT; beta-blocker for HTN emergency Intra/postoperative tachycardia/HTN
Etomidate (Amidate)	Initial: 0.3 mg/kg IV (range 0.2–0.6 mg/kg)	Moderate sedation for RSI or shoulder reduction
Fentanyl	Bolus: 1 mcg/kg. Initial: 1 mcg/kg/hr. Titrate q30min. Max: 10 mcg/kg/hr	Narcotic analgesic, sedative
Flumazenil (Romazicon)	0.2–0.5 mg IV over 30 seconds; max cumulative dose: 3 mg	Antidote for benzodiazepine overdose
Fosphenytoin sodium (Cerebyx)	Load: 15–20 phenytoin equivalents per kg by IM or IV 150 mg/min or less	Seizures
Furosemide (Lasix)	IV: 20–40 mg; PO: 20–80 mg; higher doses may be administered.	Congestive heart failure, edema, hypertension, intracranial pressure

(continued)

Medication	Dose	Use
Gentamicin sulfate ophthalmic ointment	0.5-inch ribbon to inside affected lower eyelid	Conjunctivitis and corneal abrasions
Glucagon	0.5–2 mg subcutaneous/IM/IV push	Hypoglycemia, calcium channel or beta-blocker overdose, and esophageal food bolus
Haloperidol lactate (Haldol)	Adult: 2–5 mg IM q4–8h as needed	Antipsychotic
Heparin sodium. *Check PTT and guaiac stool before giving.*	IV bolus: 60–80 unit/kg; max 4,000 units. Then 12–18 unit/kg/hr continuous infusion; follow institutional specific protocol.	Anticoagulant for acute myocardial infarction atrial fibrillation, pulmonary embolism, and stroke
Hydrocodone and acetamino-phen (Norco, Vicodin)	Adult: hydrocodone 2.5–10 mg q4–6h as needed for pain; children 2–13 years or <50 kg: hydrocodone 0.1–0.2 mg/kg/dose q4–6h, do *not* exceed six doses per day or acetaminophen max.	Opioid analgesic for pain
Ibuprofen (Motrin, Advil)	Infants >6 months and children <12 years: 10 mg/kg/dose PO (max dose 400 mg) q4–6h; max daily dose 40 mg/kg/d Children 12–17 years: 400 mg PO q4–6h; Max daily dose 2,400 mg Adults: 200–800 mg q6h as needed for pain; max daily dose 3,200 mg	Analgesic, fever, inflammation (NSAID)
Insulin (regular). *Check blood sugar every hour.*	Adult IV varies according to blood sugar: bolus (optional) 0.1 unit/kg, then IV drip according to order and blood sugar. Subcutaneously: 0.5–1 unit/kg/d divided into meal time doses.	Diabetic ketoacido-sis; hyperglycemia

(*continued*)

Medication	Dose	Use
Ipratropium bromide (Atrovent)	Child: 125–250 mcg by nebulizer q4–6h. Adult: 500 mcg by nebulizer QID. Max: 24 doses in 24 hours	Bronchodilator/ anticholinergic for asthma and chronic obstructive pulmonary disease
Labetalol hydrochloride (Normodyne)	10–20 mg IV over 2 minutes, may double dose q10–15min as often as necessary; max cumulative dose 300 mg.	Hypertension
Levalbuterol hydrochloride (Xopenex)	Nebulizer: Children 6–11 years: 0.31–0.63 mg. Children ≥12 years and adult: 0.63–2.5 mg	Bronchodilator for asthma. Causes less tachycardia than albuterol.
Levofloxacin (Levaquin). *If given too fast causes arrhythmias.*	250–750 mg by PO/IV infusion at 500 mg/hr or 750 mg over 1.5 hours	Antibiotic
Lidocaine hydrochloride (Xylocaine)	IV push: 1–1.5 mg/kg, may repeat at 0.5–0.75 mg/kg in 5–10 minutes. Intravenous drip 1–4 mg/min. ET: 2–4 mg/kg	Ventricular fibrillation/ ventricular tachycardia. Can be given subcutaneously locally to numb a wound. Comes in 1% or 2% vials.
Lidocaine with epinephrine. *Not for finger/nose/ ears/toes*	Subcutaneously locally 1% or 2% vials	To numb a bleeding wound
Lorazepam (Ativan)	0.1 mg/kg up to 4 mg IV or IM; 2–4 mg PO	Seizures, anxiety, and sedation
Magnesium sulfate	Cardiac arrest: 1–2 g in 10 mL D_5W or NS over 1–2 minutes. If stable: 1 g/50 mL NS over 30 minutes intravenously	Torsades de pointes, hypomagnesemia, preeclampsia, and asthma; smooth muscle relaxant

(continued)

Medication	Dose	Use
Mannitol strengths: 5%, 10%, 15%, 20%, and 25%	0.25–1 g/kg over 30–60 minutes; use inline filter	Intracranial pressure
Meperidine hydrochloride (Demerol),	Adult: 50–100 mg PO, IM, or IV	Opioid analgesic and shiver control
Methotrexate. Use chemotherapy precautions.	Adult: 50 mg/m² by IM	Miscarriages/ ectopic pregnancy
Methylprednisolone (Solu-Medrol)	Adult 100–250 mg IV or IM (average 125 mg)	Steroid to decrease inflammation in asthma; allergic reaction; shock
Metoprolol (Lopressor)	IV: 2.5–5 mg q2–5min (max total dose: 15 mg in 15 minutes)	Blood pressure, afib/ flutter, SVT, and ventricular rate control
Midazolam (Versed)	Initial intravenous drip: 1 mg/hr. Titrate 1 mg/hr q15min to achieve sedation goal. Max: 10 mg/hr	Moderate sedation, sedation for mechanically ventilated, or RSI
Morphine sulfate	2–5 mg IV over 1–5 minutes	Chest pain or pain (opioid analgesic)
Naloxone hydrochloride (Narcan)	IV, IM, SQ: 0.4–2 mg. Max. 10 mg in 10 minutes. Can give via ET tube or nebulizer.	Opiate overdose with respiratory or neurodepression
Nicardipine (Cardene)	IV initial: 2.5–5 mg/hr; titrate q15min to goal blood pressure; max: 15 mg/hr	Blood pressure
Nitroglycerin (Nitro-Dur, Nitrostat). *Monitor blood pressure for hypotension; must have intravenous access before giving.*	IV intial: 5–20 mcg/min titrate for chest pain/blood pressure by 5 mcg/min q3–5min. Max: 400 mcg/ min. Sublingual: one tab q5min for a 3-tablet maximum per blood pressure/chest pain	Vasodilator; chest pain; acute myocardial infarction; congestive heart failure; and hypertension

(*continued*)

Medication	Dose	Use
Nitroprusside sodium (Nipride). *Medicine reacts to light; cover material provided from pharmacy.*	IV: 0.3–2 mcg/kg/min titrate up every few minutes until stable blood pressure/chest pain	Hypertension; reduce afterload in congestive heart failure; pulmonary edema; or valve regurgitation
Norepinephrine bitartrate (Levophed)	Adult: 0.1–1 mcg/kg/min titrate to goal BP	Vasopressor for severe shock, drug overdose, or poison-induced hypotension
Oxycodone and acetaminophen (Percocet)	PO: 2.5–10 mg	Opioid analgesic
Phenytoin sodium (Dilantin). *Infiltration = tissue necrosis, be careful.*	Loading dose: 15–20 mg/kg or 1,000 mg IV. *No faster* than 50 mg/min or 20 mg/min in geriatrics.	Seizures. *Attach a micron filter.*
Promethazine hydrochloride (Phenergan)	12.5–25 mg by PO, IM, IV, or suppository	Nausea and vomiting
Proparacaine hydrochloride (Alcaine)	One to two drops to affected eye	To numb the eye. *If used repeatedly, can be corrosive to eye!*
Propofol (Diprivan)	Initial IV dose: 5 mcg/kg/min. Titrate 5 mcg/kg/min q5min Max: 50 mcg/kg/min	Sedation for mechanically ventilated, RSI. *Note:* Check state law for RN administration conditions.
Propranolol hydrochloride (Inderal)	Adult: 10–40 mg PO BID–QID. Intravenous bolus: 1–3 mg at 1 mg/min; may repeat in 2 minutes.	Hypertension; acute myocardial infarction; dysrhythmias, or thyroid storm

(continued)

Medication	Dose	Use
RhoGAM injection	Adult: 300 mcg by injection	Rh-negative pregnant mother
Sodium bicarbonate	IV bolus: 1 mEq/kg 1 amp = 50 mEq	Acidosis; hyperkalemia; diabetic ketoacidosis; lactic acidosis, and metabolic acidosis
Sodium polystyrene sulfonate (Kayexalate)	15–60 g PO or rectally	Removes potassium from body.
Succinyl-choline (Anectine)	IV: 1.5 mg/kg	Paralytic for intubation. Have ambu bag ready! Causes hyperkalemia and bradycardia.
Tenecteplase (TNKase)	Weight-based dosing; IV bolus 30–50 mg	Thrombolytic (clot buster); STEMI
Tetracaine eyedrops	One to two drops to affected eye	Topical anesthetic to the eye. *Repeated use = eye corrosion!*
Vasopressin (Pitressin)	IV/intraosseous drip: 0.03 units/min. No titration	Vasodilatory shock; catecholamine sparing vasopressor
Verapamil hydrochloride	Intravenous bolus: 5–10 mg over 3 minutes. May repeat at 10 mg q30min. Max total dose: 20 mg	PSVT with narrow complex. A-fib or A-flutter
Warfarin sodium (Coumadin, Jantoven)	Initial: 2.5–5 mg/d; titrate based on INR levels.	Anticoagulant

Note: The definitions of abbreviations can be found in Appendix D.

Appendix C
Critical Intravenous Drips

Fill out formulary kept in your hospital; keep this list in your pocket or with your calculator.

Epinephrine _____mg/_____mL (_____mcg/mL); range: 0.1 to 0.5 mcg/kg/min

Norepinephrine (Levophed) _____mg/_____mL (_____mcg/mL); range: 0.1 to 1 mcg/kg/min

Dopamine _____mg/_____mL (_____mcg/mL); initial: 5 mcg/kg/min; max = 20 mcg/kg/min

Propofol (Diprivan) _____mcg/mL; initial: 5 to 10 mcg/kg/min; max: 50 mcg/kg/min

Lidocaine _____G/_____mL (_____mcg/mL); range: 1 to 4 mg/min

Heparin _____units/_____mL (_____units/mL); weight-based hospital-specific protocol

Nitroglycerin _____mg/_____mL (_____mcg/mL); initial: 5 mcg/min; max = 400 mcg/min

Dobutamine _____mg/_____mL (_____mcg/mL); initial: 2.5 mcg/kg/min; max: 40 mcg/kg/min

Nitroprusside (Nipride) _____mg/_____mL (_____mcg/mL); initial: 0.3 to 0.5 mcg/kg/min; max = 2 mcg/kg/min

Amiodarone _____mg/_____mL (_____mg/mL); loading dose: 150 mg over 10 minutes; maintenance dose: 1 mg/min for 6 hours, then 0.5 mg/min for 18 hours

Milrinone _____mg/_____mL (_____mcg/mL); range: 0.375 to 0.75 mcg/kg/min

Midazolam (Versed) _____mg/_____mL (1 mg/___mL); range: 0.02 to 0.1 mg/kg/hr or 1 to 10 mg/hr

Labetalol _____mg/_____mL (_____mg/mL); initial: 2 mg/min; max cumulative total dose: 300 mg

Diltiazem (Cardizem) _____mg/_____mL (_____mg/mL); initial: 5 mg/hr; max: 15 mg/hr

Vasopressin _____units/_____mL (_____units/mL); fixed rate: 0.03 units/min for shock

Fentanyl _____mg/_____mL (_____mcg/mL); range: 1 to 10 mcg/kg/hr

Nicardipine (Cardene) _____mg/_____mL (_____mg/mL); initial: 5 mg/hr; max: 15 mg/hr

Appendix D
Abbreviations

The A&E nurse must be familiar with many abbreviations, which allow for quicker oral and written communication. The following is a list of abbreviations for commonly used terms in the A&E. Some acronyms are used in this text, and others are helpful in the A&E setting.

abd	abdominal
ABCs	airway, breathing, and circulation
ABG	arterial blood gas
ACLS	advanced cardiovascular life support
ACS	acute chest syndrome
ADH	antidiuretic hormone
A-fib	atrial fibrillation
A-flutter	atrial flutter
AIDS	acquired immunodeficiency syndrome
ALI	acute lung injury
alpha-PVP	alpha-pyrrolidinopentiophenone
ALT/SGPT	alanine aminotransferase/serum glutamic pyruvic transaminase
AMA	against medical advice
AMI	acute myocardial infarction
AMS	acute mountain sickness
ARDS	acute respiratory distress syndrome
ASAP	as soon as possible
ASD	atrial septal defect
AST/SGOT	aspartate aminotransferase/serum glutamic-oxaloacetic transaminase
ATP	adenosine triphosphate
AV	atrioventricular
AVSD	atrioventricular septal defect

BCEN	Board Certified Emergency Nurse
BEFAST	balance, eyes, face, arm, speech, and time
BHB	beta-hydroxybutyrate
BHO	butane honey oil
b.i.d.	twice daily
BiPAP	bilevel positive airway pressure
BMP	basic metabolic panel
BNP	brain-type natriuretic peptide
BP	blood pressure
bpm	beats per minute
BRAT	bananas, rice, applesauce, and toast
BS	blood sugar
BSC	bedside commode
BUN	blood urea nitrogen
BVM	bag valve mask
CAB	circulation, airway, and breathing
CAD	coronary artery disease
CBC	complete blood count
CDC	Centers for Disease Control and Prevention
CEN	certified emergency nurse
CHD	congenital heart disease
CHF	congestive heart failure
CKMB	creatine kinase MB
CMP	complete metabolic panel
CO_2	carbon dioxide
c/o	complaining of
COPD	chronic obstructive pulmonary disease
COVID-19	coronavirus disease 2019
CP	chest pain
C-PAP	continuous positive airway pressure
CPI	Crisis Prevention Institute
CVP	central venous pressure
CPR	cardiopulmonary resuscitation
CSF	cerebrospinal fluid
CT	computed tomography
CVA	cerebrovascular accident
D5W	dextrose 5% in water
DAI	drug assisted intubation
DC	discharge
DDAVP	desmopressin acetate
DIB	difficulty in breathing
DIC	disseminated intravascular coagulation
DKA	diabetic ketoacidosis
DNR	do not resuscitate
dx	diagnose
ECMO	extracorporeal membrane oxygenation
ED	emergency department
EKG	electrocardiogram
ELISA	enzyme-linked immunosorbent assay

EMTALA	Emergency Medical Treatment and Active Labor Act
ENA	Emergency Nurses Association
ENPC	emergency nurse pediatric course
ENT	ear, nose, and throat
ER	emergency room
ERCP	endoscopic retrograde cholangiopancreatography
ESI	Emergency Severity Index
ET	endotracheal tube
ETOH	alcohol
FAST	focused assessment with sonography in trauma
FEMA	Federal Emergency Management Agency
FFP	fresh frozen plasma
FHT	fetal heart tones
FO	foreign object
G & C	gonorrhea and chlamydia
GCS	Glasgow Coma Scale
GERD	gastroesophageal reflux disease
GHB	gamma-hydroxybutyric acid
GI	gastrointestinal
gtts	drops
GYN	gynecological
HA	headache
HACE	high-altitude cerebral edema
HAI	high-altitude illness
HAPE	high-altitude pulmonary edema
HCO_3^-	bicarbonate
H_2CO_3	carbonic acid
Hcg	human chorionic gonadotropin
HCT	hematocrit
HELLP	hemolytic anemia, elevated liver enzymes, and low platelet count
HGB	hemoglobin
H & H	hemoglobin and hematocrit
HHNC	hyperosmolar, hyperglycemic nonketotic coma
HHS	hyperosmolar hyperglycemic syndrome
HIV	human immunodeficiency virus
HOB	head of the bed
HPV	human papillomavirus
HTN	hypertension
hx	history
IBS	irritable bowel syndrome
ICP	increased cranial pressure
ICU	intensive care unit
I&D	incision and drainage
IM	intramuscular
IMR	intermediate restorative material
IN	intranasal
INR	international normalized ratio
IO	intraosseous
I&O	intake and output
IUP	intrauterine pregnancy
IV	intravenous
IVC	inferior vena cava
JVD	jugular vein distention

LFT	liver function test
LLQ	left lower quadrant
LMWH	low molecular weight heparin
LOC	loss of consciousness
LP	lumbar puncture
LSD	D-lysergic acid diethylamide
LUQ	left upper quadrant
LWBS	left without being seen
MDI	meter dose inhaler
MDMA	3,4-methylenedioxy-methamphetamine
MERS	Middle Eastern respiratory syndrome
MRSA	methicillin-resistant *Staphylococcus aureus*
MS	multiple sclerosis
MVI	multivitamin
NAC	N-acetylcysteine
NC	nasal cannula
Neb	nebulizer
NG	nasogastric
NHTRC	National Human Trafficking Resource Center
NIHSS	National Institutes of Health Stroke Scale
NINDS	National Institute for Neurological Disorders and Stroke
NPO	nothing by mouth
NPS	new psychoactive substance
NRB	nonrebreather
NRP	Neonatal Resuscitation Program
NS	normal saline
NSAID	nonsteroidal anti-inflammatory drug
NTG	nitroglycerine
NV	nausea and vomiting
NVD	nausea/vomiting/diarrhea
O_2	oxygen
OB	Obstetrical
OD	overdose
OM	otitis media
OR	operating room
os	opening
2-PAM	pralidoxime
$PaCO_2$	partial pressure of carbon dioxide
PALS	pediatric advanced life support
PAT	pediatric assessment triangle
PCC	prothrombin complex concentrate
PCP	phencyclidine
PCT	procalcitonin
PDA	patent ductus arteriosus
PE	pulmonary embolism
PEA	pulseless electrical activity
PEEP	positive end-expiratory pressure
PID	pelvic inflammatory disease
PIH	pregnancy-induced hypertension
PLT	platelets
PO	by mouth

PPE	personal protective equipment
pr	by rectum
PRBC	packed red blood cells
prn	as needed
PSI	per square inch
PSVT	paroxysmal supraventricular tachycardia
pt.	patient
PT	prothrombin time
PTT	partial thromboplastin time
PTU	propylthiouracil
PVC	premature ventricular contraction
PVD	peripheral vascular disease
RBBB	right bundle branch block
RBC	red blood cell
REBOA	resuscitative endovascular balloon occlusion
resp	respiratory
RF	renal failure
RL	Ringer's lactate
RLQ	right lower quadrant
ROM	range of motion
RSI	rapid sequence intubation
RSV	respiratory syncytial virus
RUQ	right upper quadrant
SANE	sexual assault nurse examiner
SARS	severe acute respiratory syndrome
SC	subcutaneous
SDS	safety data sheets
SIADH	syndrome of inappropriate antidiuretic hormone
SIDS	sudden infant death syndrome
SIRS	systemic inflammatory response syndrome
SL	under the tongue
SOB	shortness of breath
SQ	subcutaneous
s/s	signs and symptoms
stat	immediately
STEMI	ST-segment elevated myocardial infarction
STI	sexually transmitted infection
SVT	supraventricular tachycardia
SZ	seizure
TB	tuberculosis
TBSA	total burn surface area
TCA	tricyclic antidepressants
Tdap	tetanus diphtheria and pertussis
TIA	transient ischemic attack
TNCC	trauma nurse core course
tPA	tissue plasminogen activator (alteplase)
TSS	toxic shock syndrome
TTM	targeted temperature management
Tx	treat or treatment
UA	urinalysis
US	ultrasound

UTI	urinary tract infection
VF	ventricular fibrillation
VOC	vaso-occlusive crisis
VS	vital signs
VSD	ventricular septal defect
VT	ventricular tachycardia
WBC	white blood cell

Appendix E
12-Lead EKGs and
Common Dysrhythmias

PROPER EKG LEAD PLACEMENT

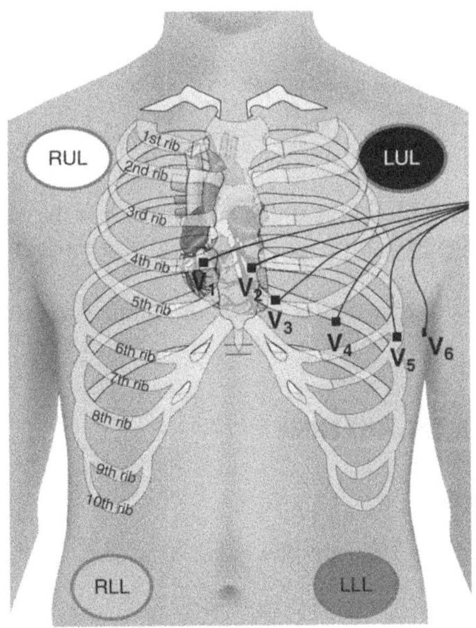

Limb leads may be placed symmetrically on the upper and lower extremities on a nonbony surface.

BREAKDOWN OF NORMAL SINUS RHYTHM

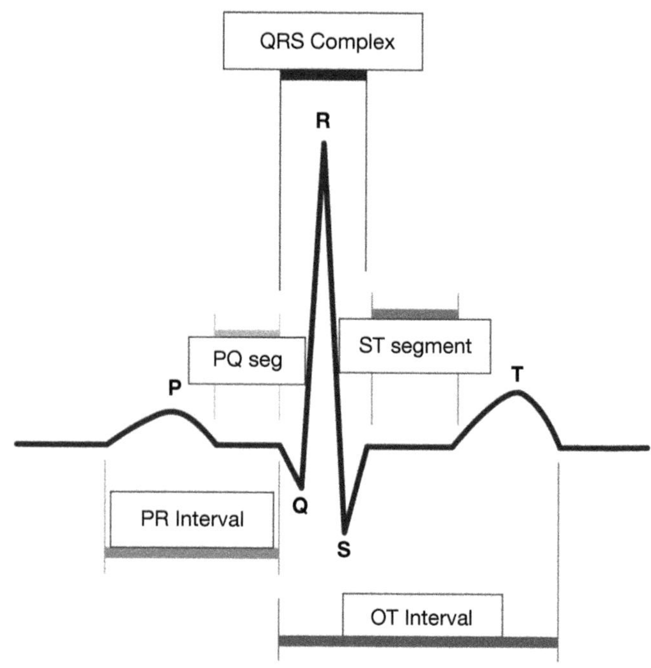

P wave represents: contraction and depolarization of the atria.

QRS complex represents contraction and depolarization of the ventricles.

T wave represents ventricular relaxation, repolarization, and passive filling.

OTHER COMMON EKG RHYTHMS

Normal Sinus Rhythm

Note P wave for every QRS complex. Rate is regular.

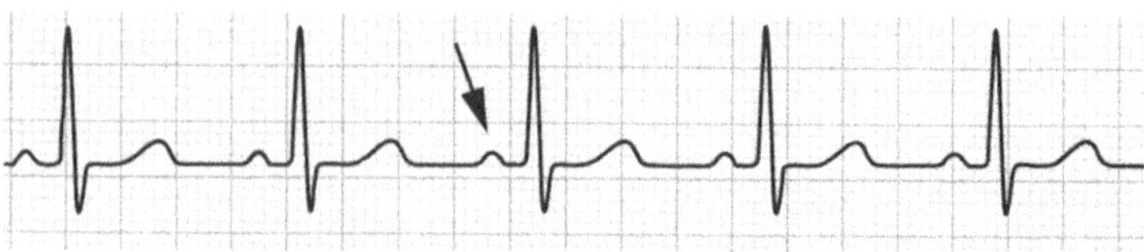

Atrial Fibrillation

Note atrial rhythm waves, P wave unidentifiable, and irregular rate.

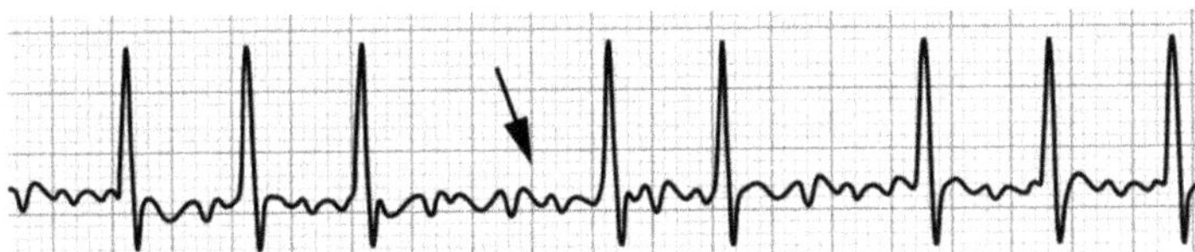

Atrial Flutter

Note multiple-peaked or saw-tooth-like P waves.

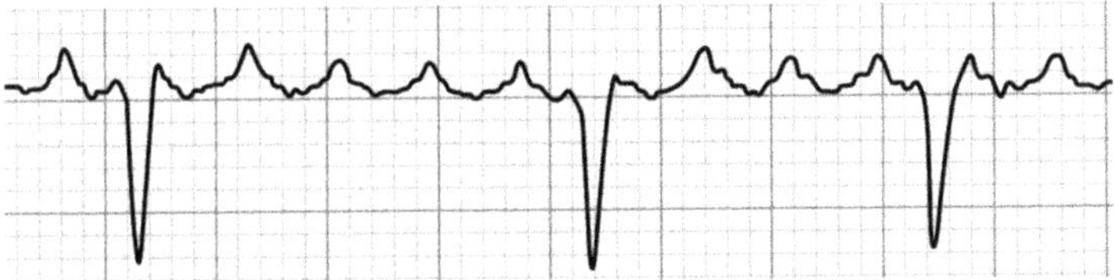

Left Bundle Branch Block

Note wide QRS >0.12 seconds.

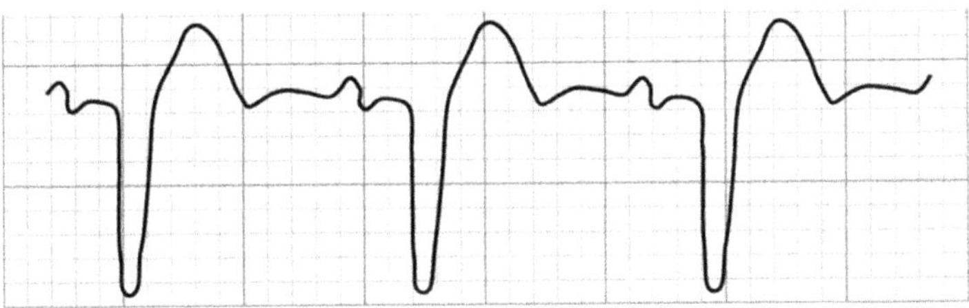

First-Degree Block

Note rate is regular and the PR interval is longer or >0.20 seconds. If the R is far from P, it might be first degree.

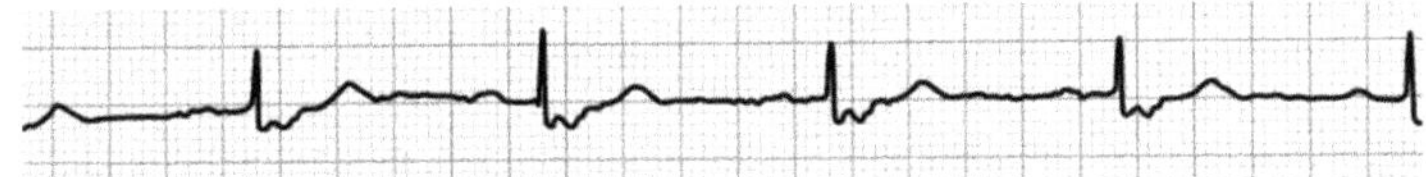

Second-Degree Heart Block, Mobitz Type I, or Wenckebach

Note irregular yet patterned rate. See how PR interval becomes progressively longer until finally a QRS complex is dropped.

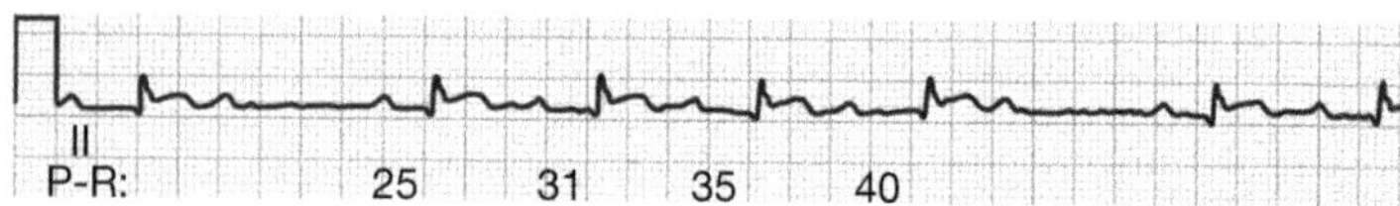

Essential Facts

To remember Wenckebach, think Wenke, Wenke Wenke Bach.... The PR interval is long, longer, longer, dropped.

Second-Degree Heart Block, Mobitz Type II

The PR interval does not progressively lengthen, but a QRS complex gets dropped regularly.

Essential Facts

If the rhythm is regularly missing a Q, it might be Mobitz 2.

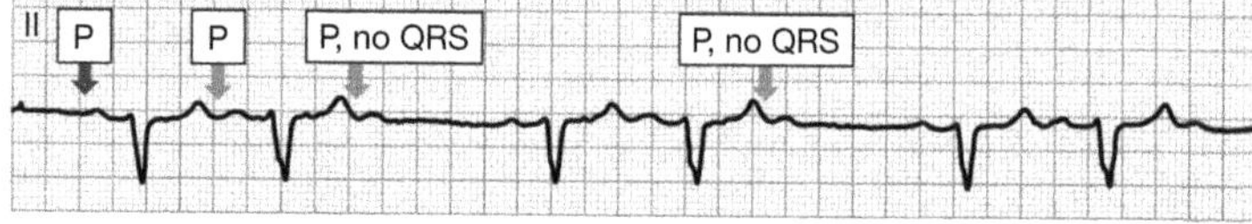

Third-Degree or (Complete) Heart Block

The P waves occur at regular intervals and the QRS complexes occur at regular intervals but they are disconnected and do not occur together. This is due to a complete electrical blockage between the atria (p wave) and the ventricles (QRS complex).

Essential Facts

If the Ps and Qs don't agree, it is probably third degree.

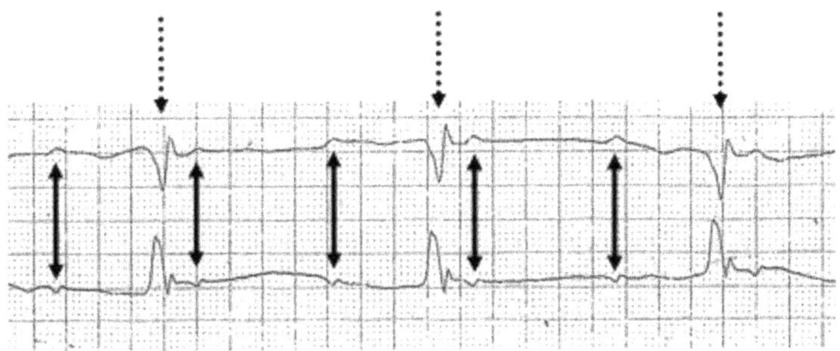

Paced or Ventricular-Paced Rhythm

Note pacer spikes instead of P waves.

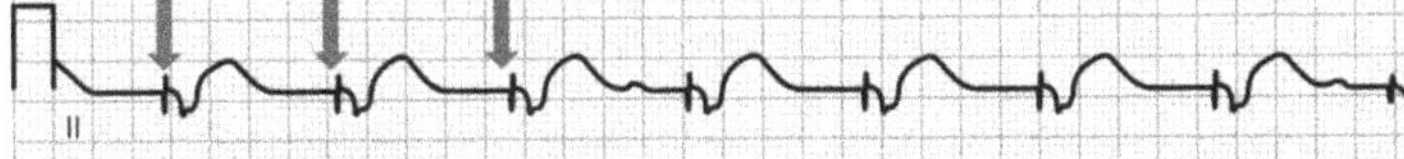

Wolff-Parkinson-White Syndrome

Note the delta wave in the upstroke of the QRS complex.

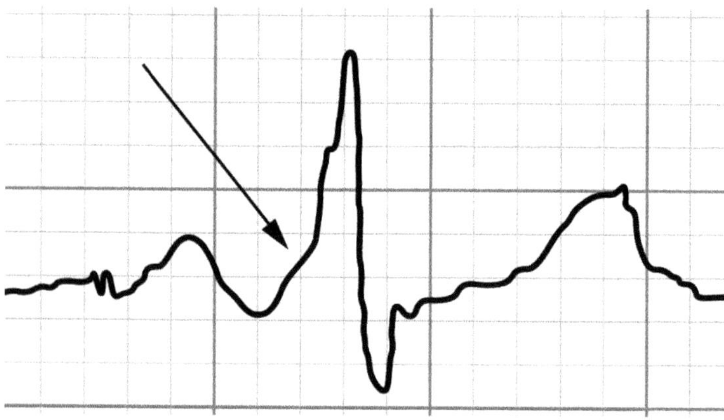

Torsades de Pointes

Torsades de pointes is French for "turning or twisting of the points." Note that this particular type of ventricular tachycardia turns or twists on its axis much like a strand of DNA. The treatment for this type of tachycardia is magnesium sulfate.

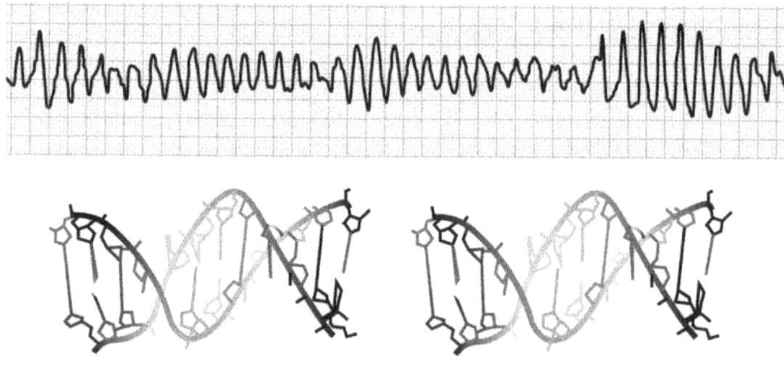

Junctional

Note there are either no P waves present or the P waves are inverted.

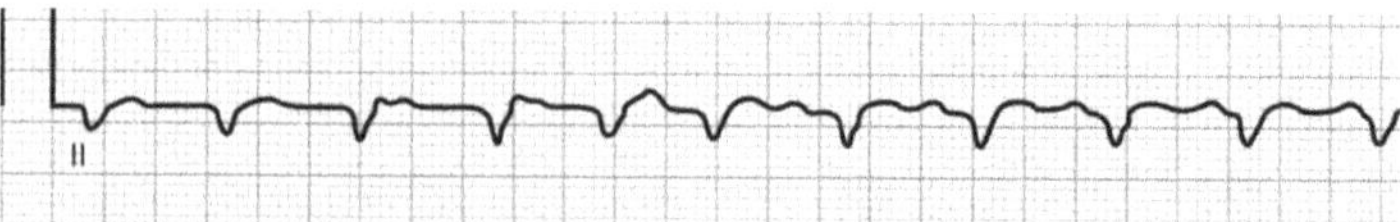

Premature Atrial Contraction

Note that the underlying rate is regular except for an occasional early narrow complex beat.

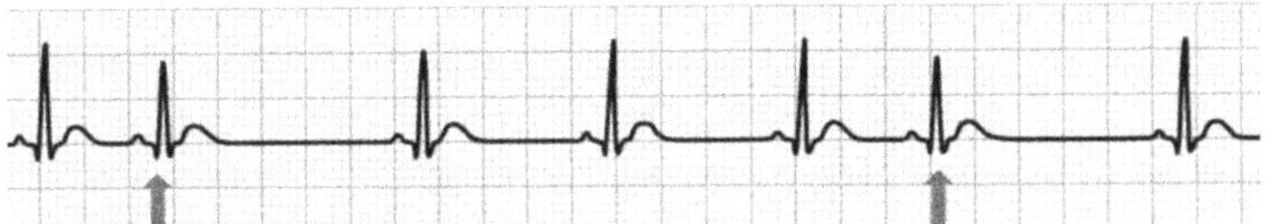

Premature Ventricular Contraction

Note that the underlying rate is regular with an occasional wide complex beat.

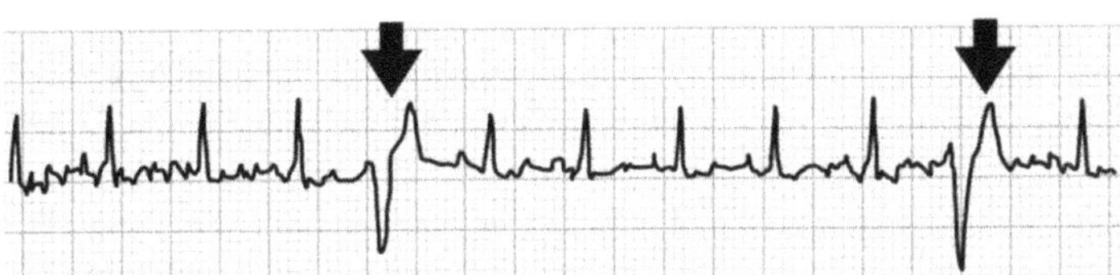

Bigeminy

Note the premature ventricular contraction (PVC) with every other beat.

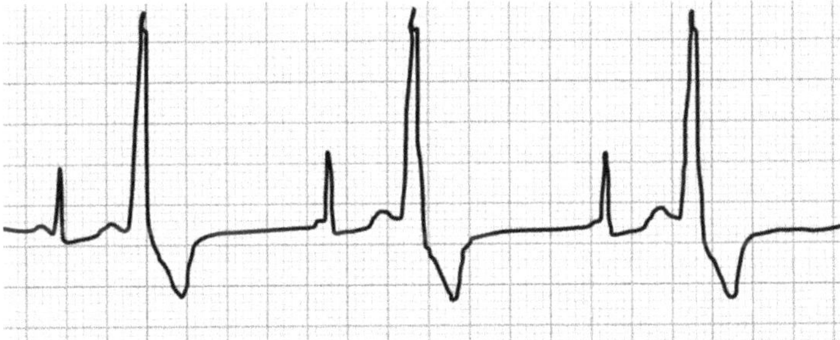

Couplet

Note two PVCs in a row.

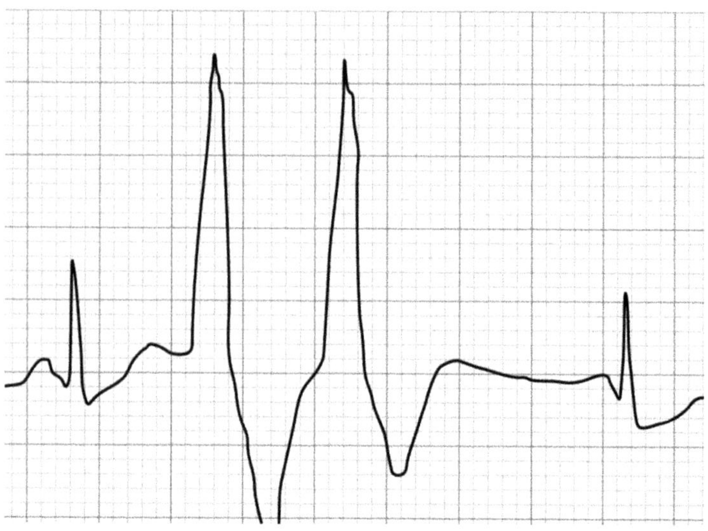

Appendix F
Skills Check-Off Sheets

Administrative Checklist

Employee Name _______________________

Start Date _______________________

Administrative Checklist Items	Verbally Reviewed	Physically Performed	Educator's Initials
Call-in policy			
Clock-in/clock-out procedures			
Communication books and boards			
Computer down time backup procedures			
Computer systems access/sign-up for classes			
Certifications on file:			
■ License verification			
■ Basic life support (BLS)			
■ Advanced cardiac life support (ACLS)			
■ Pediatric advanced life support (PALS)			

(continued)

Administrative Checklist Items	Verbally Reviewed	Physically Performed	Educator's Initials
■ National Institutes of Health Stroke Scale (NIHSS)			
■ Crisis Prevention Institute (CPI; Nonviolent Crisis Intervention)			
■ Other:			
Discuss orientation needs and establish goals			
Dress code			
Education resources/requirements/ opportunities			
Employee injury incident reports			
Emergency management codes			
■ Code Blue			
■ Fire			
■ Security			
■ Sepsis			
■ Severe Weather			
■ Shooting			
■ Stroke			
■ Electrical or water			
■ Missing infant			
■ Missing person			
■ Hazmat			
■ Disaster			
■ Bomb threat			
Email setup and access			
Emergency Medical Treatment and Active Labor Act (EMTALA) guidelines			
Evacuation plan, emergency exits			

(continued)

Administrative Checklist Items	Verbally Reviewed	Physically Performed	Educator's Initials
Evaluation form, reassess goals weekly			
Fire extinguishers and pull stations			
Intercom/patient call light system			
Job description signed and filed			
Latex allergy protocol and procedures			
Manual time record			
Medical gas shutoffs			
Medication adverse reaction form or procedure			
Nursing documentation forms			
Nursing/A&E policy and procedures manual			
Orient to unit/staff personnel/registration			
Orientation forms and packet			
Orientation schedule			
Patient-appropriate room assignments			
Patient assignment board procedures			
Patient belongings left in department			
Patient education resources			
Patient flow in department			
Patient incident report			
Policy, protocols, and procedures manual database			
Professional advancement opportunities			
Reference tools			
■ Medications			
■ Intravenous (IV) compatibility charts			
Patient education			

(continued)

Administrative Checklist Items	Verbally Reviewed	Physically Performed	Educator's Initials
Patient rights			
Registration process			
Safety data sheets (SDS)			
Scavenger hunt			
Schedule/request form for time off/ paid time off (PTO)			
Service recovery			
Sick call procedure			
Staffing assignments			
Staff meetings			
Storeroom supplies			
Supply stocking procedure			
Telephone system			
Time and attendance policy			
Tour of department			
Videos/online learning			
Workplace violence policy			

Preceptor Skills Checklist

Employee Name_______________________

Start Date_______________________

Skill Item	Verbally Reviewed	Physically Performed	Preceptor's Initials
Abuse/neglect evaluation			
Admission procedure			
Advance directives and consent for do-not-resuscitate (DNR) status			
Airway open and maintained: jaw thrust or head tilt chin lift			
Airway devices: oral and nasal airways measurements/insertions			
Alcohol withdrawal assessment			
Anaphylaxis procedures			
Anesthesia consent			
Animal bite protocols			
Arterial blood gas interpretation			
Assistance notification: ■ Adult protective services ■ Supervisor ■ Security, law enforcement ■ Chaplain ■ Division of family and children services ■ Case/risk management/ethics committee			
Bag valve mask: adult, pediatric, neonate			
Bladder irrigations			
Blood work interpretation			
Blood/blood products administration and consent forms			
Burn care procedures (Major and Minor)			
Cardiac arrhythmias			

(continued)

Skill Item	Verbally Reviewed	Physically Performed	Preceptor's Initials
Cardiac monitoring systems central, portable, and bedside			
Cardiopulmonary arrest nursing roles			
Central line care and dressing application			
Central port access (gripper/Huber needle)			
Central vein access kit and procedures			
Chest tube equipment/procedures: hemo/pneumothorax			
Code blue forms and code blue critique form			
Code blue procedure in the A&E			
Code blue procedures outside of the A&E			
Crash cart use procedures, checks			
Crutches return demonstration and documentation			
Cricothyrotomy kit and procedure			
C-spine collars immobilization and removal techniques			
Death in the department			
Deceased patient data documentation form			
Decontamination equipment			
Defibrillator/pacer procedures			
Dental repair equipment or referrals			
Diabetic ketoacidosis (DKA) protocol			
Difficult people, working with them			
Disaster response plan			
Discharge procedures and instructions			

(continued)

Skill Item	Verbally Reviewed	Physically Performed	Preceptor's Initials
Documentation ■ Assessments 　▪ Triage 　▪ Primary 　▪ Secondary 　▪ Focused 　▪ Discharge ■ Interventions ■ Medication ■ Outcomes ■ Pain ■ Patient education			
Doppler: vessel and obstetric uses			
Ear irrigation procedure			
EKG 12-lead check-off and interpretation			
End title CO_2 monitoring, devices, and documentation			
Emergency medications and resource tools			
Emergency medical services (EMS) radio and H.E.A.R. system radio			
Endotracheal intubation and rapid-sequence intubation			
Eye exams supplies: Wood's lamp, eye kit, slit lamp, fluorescein strips			
Eye irrigation techniques			
Fall precautions, policy, and documentation			
Fetal heart monitoring in A&E			
Fracture reduction assist			
Gastric lavage			
Gastric tubes (oral/nasal) insertions and setup			
Gastrointestinal (GI) bleed procedures			
Glucose-monitoring meter and documentation			

(continued)

382

Skill Item	Verbally Reviewed	Physically Performed	Preceptor's Initials
Hand hygiene			
Handoff report and bedside shift report			
Head lamp (ear, nose, and throat [ENT]) uses and location			
Hemostatic dressings to control bleeding			
Heimlich valve pneumothorax kit			
High risk/behavior patient care procedures, policy, and documentation			
Holding of admitted patients			
Imaging diagnostic tests ■ x-ray ■ CT scan ■ MRI ■ Ventilation/perfusion (VQ) scan ■ Ultrasound (US) ■ Interventional radiology			
Incision and drainage procedures			
Infusion protocols (cardiac/emergency infusions)			
Instrument recycling (disposable/non-disposable)			
IV infusion and patient-controlled analgesia (PCA) pump			
IV insertion intermittent needle therapy (INT) procedures			
Joint commission preparedness information			
Laceration repair tray, staples, sutures, skin glue			
Language translation methods (verbal/written)			
Left against medical advice (AMA) or left without being seen (LWBS) procedures			
Left without treatment procedures			

(continued)

Skill Item	Verbally Reviewed	Physically Performed	Preceptor's Initials
Lumbar puncture tray, spinal needles, procedure/patient position			
Medication administration policies and procedures ■ Intravenous (IV) ■ Intramuscular (IM) ■ By Mouth (PO) ■ Intranasal (IN) ■ Intraosseous (IO) ■ Subcutaneous (SQ) ■ Respiratory aerosol nebulizer			
Medication reconciliation documentation			
Methotrexate administration for ectopic pregnancy			
Minors in the A&E: Legal policies and procedures			
Miscarriage (complete/incomplete) referrals before 20 weeks (Rachel's Gift)/after 20 weeks			
N95 mask fit test size			
Nasal trays, tampons			
Needle decompression for tension pneumothorax			
Neonate patient care			
Neurologic assessment/documentation			
Neurologist consult			
Neutropenia policy and procedures			
Nosebleed procedures and equipment			
Obstetrical (OB) exam/specimens and products of conception			
OB precipitous delivery procedures and supplies			
OB trauma patient care			

(continued)

Skill Item	Verbally Reviewed	Physically Performed	Preceptor's Initials
Operating room (OR) admission and preoperative checklist			
Orthopedic finger traps			
Panic buttons			
Pain management policy/procedures			
Patient priority setting and acuity assignment			
Patient transfer procedure, forms, and documentation			
Pediatric broselow cart checks, procedures			
Pediatric care tools and references			
Pediatric positioning and securing (papoose board)			
Pelvic exam supplies, equipment, and stretchers			
Pericardiocentesis tray			
Peritoneal lavage			
Pervenous temporary pacemaker			
Phlebotomy checkoff, venipunctures lab, and IV access			
pH paper use and documentation			
Poison control notification/ documentation			
Personal protective equipment (PPE) donning and doffing procedures			
Precautions:			
■ Airborne			
■ Contact			
■ C-Diff contact enteric precautions			
■ Droplet			

(continued)

Skill Item	Verbally Reviewed	Physically Performed	Preceptor's Initials
RhoGAM/blood product administration			
Safe room preparation, removal of contraband			
Seclusion/restraint policy behavioral and medical			
Security policy regarding behavioral health patients			
Sedation and analgesia policy and procedures/forms			
Seizure precautions and patient care			
Sepsis screening and protocol			
Sexual assault/rape examination procedure and protocol			
Soiled utility room procedures and uses			
Specimen collections			
■ Respiratory syncytial virus specimen collection (RSV)			
■ Rapid Strep Screen			
■ Sputum			
■ Flu			
■ Nasopharyngeal (COVID-19)			
■ Stool			
■ Hemoccult/stool/gastric specimen collection			
■ Urine ■ Urine pregnancy			
Splint application and documentation ■ Synthetic (Orthoglass) ■ Velcro ■ Hare traction			

(continued)

Skill Item	Verbally Reviewed	Physically Performed	Preceptor's Initials
ST-segment elevated myocardial infarction (STEMI) or chest pain protocol ■ Cath lab procedure ■ Alteplase for STEMI			
Stroke protocol administration of alteplase or thrombectomy			
Substance abuse withdrawal scales			
Suicidal/homicidal forms			
Surgical consent			
Suture/staple removal procedure			
Swallow or dysphagia screening			
Therapeutic hypothermia or targeted temperature management protocol			
Tourniquets, military grade (stop the bleed)			
Tracheostomy tray and procedure and documentation			
Transcutaneous pacemaker procedure and documentation			
Trauma roles and responsibilities			
Transport of critical ICU or telemetry patient			
Triage guidelines/protocols (disaster and non-disaster)			
Triage travel and infection screening			
Ultrasound portable and nonportable procedures			
Urinary catheterization procedures			
■ Intermittent catheter			
■ Indwelling			

(continued)

Skill Item	Verbally Reviewed	Physically Performed	Preceptor's Initials
■ External female catheter			
■ Condom catheter			
Urine strainer			
Urology consult, cart/supplies			
Vaccines procedures and documentation ■ Tetanus ■ Rabies			
Ventilator troubleshooting and patient care			
Visual acuity (adult or pediatric) Snellen chart			
Vital sign monitoring and documentation			
Warming devices			
■ External warming device/blanket			
■ IV or internal warming			
■ Infant			
Worker's compensation drug screening			

Complete post-orientation evaluation form, assessment of the clinical orientation process, review goals, and assess need for orientation extension.

Preceptor Name/Initials: _______________________
Preceptor Signature: __________________________

Employee Signature: __________________________
Orientation End Date: _________________________

Bibliography

American Heart Association. (2020). *Advanced cardiovascular life support.* American Heart Association.

American Heart Association. (2020). *Pediatric advanced life support.* American Heart Association.

American Heart Association. (2018). Target: Stroke. https://www.stroke .org/-/media/files/professional/quality-improvement/target-stroke/ target-stroke-phase-iii/aha-qi-target-stroke-phase-3-brochure.pdf

American Medical Association. (2012). *Basic disaster life support version 3.0.* American Medical Association.

Armstrong, J. H., & Schwartz, R. B. (2011). *Advanced disaster life support version 3.0.* American Medical Association.

Association of Women's Health, Obstetric, and Neonatal Nurses. (2018). *Postbirth warning signs education program.* Association of Women's Health, Obstetric, and Neonatal Nurses. https://www.awhonn.org/wp -content/uploads/2020/02/pbwssylhandoutenglish.pdf

Basile, J., & Bloch, M. J. (2014, November 18). Overview of hypertension in adults. http://www.uptodate.com/contents/overview-of-hypertension-in -adults?source=search_result&search=hypertension&selectedTitle=1~150

Blank, F. S., Miller, M., Nichols, J., Smithline, H., Crabb, G., & Pekow, P. (2009). Blood glucose measurement in patients with suspected diabetic ketoacidosis: A comparison of Abbott MediSense PCx point-of-care meter values to reference laboratory values. *Journal of Emergency Nursing, 35,* 93–96. https://doi.org/10.1016/j.jen.2008.01.008

Bowen, P. (2016). Early identification, rapid response, and effective treatment of acute stroke: Utilizing teleneurology to ensure optimal clinical outcomes. *MEDSURG Nursing, 25*(4), 241–243.

Brecher, D. M.-B. (2020). *Insights & Innovation: Bias in triage decision making...yes, we are all guilty (Brought to you by MedNition).* ENX20 ENA National Conference. Virtual Online.

Centers for Disease Control and Prevention. (2020, February 27). Ebola (Ebola virus disease). https://www.cdc.gov/coronavirus/2019-ncov/

Centers for Disease Control and Prevention. (2019, June 27). Opioid overdose. https://www.cdc.gov/drugoverdose/epidemic/index.html

Centers for Disease Control and Prevention. (2021, February 28). Coronavirus Disease 2019 (COVID-19). https://www.cdc.gov/coronavirus/2019-ncov/

Chameides, L., Samson, R. A., Schexnayder, S. M., & Hazinski, M. F. (2016). *Pediatric advanced life support*. American Heart Association.

Derr, P., McEvoy, M., & Tardiff, J. (2014). *Emergency & critical care pocket guide* (8th ed.). Jones & Bartlett.

Dowling Dols, J.-B., Beckmann-Mendez, D.-B., McDow, J., Walker, K., & Moon, M. D.-C. (2019). Human trafficking victim identification, assessment, and intervention strategies in South Texas Emergency Departments. *Journal of Emergency Nursing, 45*(6), 622–632. https://doi.org/10.1016/j.jen.2019.07.002

Emergency Nurses Association. (2018a). *CEN review manual* (5th ed.). Jones & Bartlett.

Emergency Nurses Association. (2018b). *Emergency nursing core curriculum* (7th ed.). Elsevier.

Emergency Nurses Association. (2018c). *Emergency nursing pediatric course* (5th ed.). Emergency Nurses Association.

Emergency Nurses Association. (2018d). Position statement triage qualifications and competency. https://www.ena.org/docs/default-source/resource-library/practice-resources/position-statements/triagequalificationscompetency.pdf?sfvrsn=a0bbc268_8

Emergency Nurses Association. (2019). *Trauma nurse core course* (8th ed.). Emergency Nurses Association.

Emergency Nurses Association. (2020a). *Implementation handbook 2020 edition emergency severity index* (4th ed.). Emergency Nurses Association. https://www.ena.org/education/esi

Emergency Nurses Association. (2020b). *Sheehy's emergency nursing principles and practice* (7th ed.). Elsevier.

Emergency Nurses Association, Hammond, B. B., & Zimmermann, P. G. (Eds.). (2013). *Sheehy's manual of emergency care* (7th ed.). Elsevier Mosby.

Gasparis Vonfrolio, L. (1999). *The one and only CEN review course*. Education Enterprises.

Goldsworthy, S., & Graham, L. (2014). *Compact clinical guide to mechanical ventilation*. Springer Publishing Company.

Green, C. (2016). Human trafficking: Preparing for a unique patient population. *American Nurse Today, 11*(1), 9–12.

Gupta, A. G., & Adler, M. D. (2016). Management of an unexpected delivery in the emergency department. *Clinical Pediatric Emergency Medicine, 17*(2), 89–98. https://doi.org/10.1016/j.cpem.2016.03.002

Hamilton, R. J. (2016). *Tarascon pocket pharmacopoeia* (30th ed.). Jones & Bartlett.

Haroutunian, M., & Bono, M. J. (2014). High-altitude illness. *Emergency Medicine, 46*(5), 202–210. https://www.mdedge.com/emergencymedicine/article/82565/sports-medicine/high-altitude-illness

Harris, S. N., Garth, A. P., Spanierman, C. S., & Salas, R. N. (2018, September 18). How are animal bites characterized? https://www.medscape.com/answers/768875-60762/how-are-animal-bites-characterized

Heslin, S. M., Bronson, S. M., Feiler, M. R., Fuhrer, J. M., King, C. R.-C., Leonard, M. M., Raymundo, L. M., Rowe, A. L., & Morley, E. J. (2019). Team triage intervention, including licensed practical nurse, to increase HIV testing rates in the emergency department: A quality improvement project. *Journal of Emergency Nursing, 45*(6), 685–689. https://doi.org/10.1016/j.jen.2019.07.016

Lee, B., Ishimine, P., Joseph, M., & Mehta, S. (2017). Evaluation and treatment of minors. *Annals of Emergency Medicine, 71*(2), 225–232. https://www.sciencedirect.com/science/article/abs/pii/S0196064417 30879X

Lim, C. H. L., Turner, A., & Lim, B. X. (2016). Patching for corneal abrasion. *Cochrane Database of System Reviews, 2016*(7), CD004764.

Mader, S. S., & Windelspecht, M. (2016). *Biology* (12th ed.). McGraw-Hill.

Miller, N. J. A.-C. (2020). *Waiting to exhale—Management of life-threatening asthma.* EN20X ENA National Conference. Virtual.

Mitchell, J. (n.d.). Critical incident stress debriefing. http://www.info-trauma.org/flash/media-f/mitchellCriticalIncidentStressDebriefing.pdf

National Institutes of Health. (2014, September 8). *Evidence-based management of sickle cell disease: Expert Panel Report, 2014.* http://www.nhlbi.nih.gov/health-pro/guidelines/sickle-cell-disease-guidelines

National Sexual Violence Resource Center. (2018). *Sexual Assault Response Team Toolkit.* National Sexual Violence Resource Center. https://www.nsvrc.org/sarts/toolkit

Nevid, J. S., Rathus, S. A., & Greene, B. (2014). *Abnormal psychology* (9th ed.). Pearson.

Niermeyer, S. (2015). From the Neonatal Resuscitation Program to Helping Babies Breathe: Global impact of educational programs in neonatal resuscitation. *Seminars in Fetal and Neonatal Medicine, 20,* 300–308. https://doi.org/10.1016/j.siny.2015.06.005

Office of Public Health Preparedness and Response. (2015, November 18). Emergency preparedness and response. https://emergency.cdc.gov/bioterrorism/

Pagana, K. D., & Pagana, T. J. (2013). *St. Mosby's manual of diagnostic and laboratory tests* (11th ed.). Elsevier Mosby.

Patterson, K., Grenny, J., McMillan, R., & Switzler, A. (2011). *Crucial conversations: Tools for talking when stakes are high* (2nd ed.). McGraw-Hill Education.

Porth, C. M. (2015). *Essentials of pathophysiology* (4th ed.). Wolters Kluwer.

Prosser, J., & Nelson, L. (2012). The toxicology of bath salts: A review of synthetic cathinones. *Journal of Medical Toxicology, 8*(1), 33–42. https://doi.org/10.1007/s13181-011-0193-z

Rachel's Gift. (2021). *Recommendations for emergency departments.* Rachel's Gift. https://www.rachelsgift.org/emergency-departments.html

Sedlak, S. K. (2014). Environmental emergencies. In ENA's, B. B. Hammond, & P. S. Zimmerman (Eds.), *Sheehy's manual of emergency care* (7th ed., pp. 337–340). Elsevier.

Shepherd, S. M., & Shoff, W. H. (2014). An urban northeastern United States alligator bite. *American Journal of Emergency Medicine, 32*(5), 487.e1–487.e3. https://doi.org/10.1016/j.ajem.2013.11.004

Studer, Q. (2012). *The great employee handbook: Making work and life better.* Fire Starter Publishing.

Substance Abuse and Mental Health Services Administration. (2016). *Opioid overdose prevention toolkit.* Department of Health and Human Services, Substance Abuse and Mental Health Services Administration.

Tamkin, G. W. (2020). Cop Tox: What's new on the street. ENX20 ENA Annual Conference. Virtual Online.

Valdez, A. (2019). Who cares for the emergency nurse? *Journal of Emergency Nursing, 45*(6), 602–604. https://doi.org/10.1016/j.jen.2019.09.007

Visser, L. S., Montejano, A. S., & Grossman, V. A. (2015). *Fast facts for the triage nurse.* Springer Publishing Company.

Wang, G. S. (2019, October 22). Cannabis (marijuana): Acute intoxication. https://www.uptodate.com/contents/cannabis-marijuana-acute -intoxication

Wiegand, T. (2016). Nonsteroidal anti-inflammatory drug (NSAID) toxicity treatment & management. http://emedicine.medscape.com/article/816117 -treatment

Wolf, L. (2011). Ten Ways to Get Fooled in Triage. *12th Annual Southeastern Seaboard Emergency Nursing Symposium.* Atlanta.

Wolters Kluwer Clinical Drug Information. (2020). Lexi drugs, 2.4.0. http:// online.lexi.com/action/home

World Health Organization. (2018, November 6). Influenza seasonal. https:// www.who.int/en/news-room/fact-sheets/detail/influenza-(seasonal)

Index